Health Consequences of Service During the Persian Gulf War: Recommendations for Research and Information Systems

Committee to Review the Health Consequences of Service
During the Persian Gulf War

Medical Follow-up Agency

Institute of Medicine

NATIONAL ACADEMY PRESS
Washington, D.C. 1996

NATIONAL ACADEMY PRESS • 2101 Constitution Avenue, N.W. • Washington, D.C. 20418

NOTICE: The project that is the subject of this report was approved by the Governing Board of the National Research Council, whose members are drawn from the councils of the National Academy of Sciences, the National Academy of Engineering, and the Institute of Medicine. The members of the committee responsible for the report were chosen for their special competencies and with regard for appropriate balance.

This report has been reviewed by a group other than the authors according to procedures approved by a Report Review Committee consisting of members of the National Academy of Sciences, the National Academy of Engineering, and the Institute of Medicine.

The Institute of Medicine was chartered in 1970 by the National Academy of Sciences to enlist distinguished members of the appropriate professions in the examination of policy matters pertaining to the health of the public. In this, the Institute acts under both the Academy's 1863 congressional charter responsibility to be an adviser to the federal government and its own initiative in identifying issues of medical care, research, and education. Dr. Kenneth I. Shine is president of the Institute of Medicine.

Support for this study was provided equally by the Department of Veterans Affairs and the Department of Defense (Contract No. V101(93)P-1417).

International Standard Book No. 0-309-05536-9

Additional copies of the report are available for sale from:

National Academy Press
Box 285
2101 Constitution Avenue, N.W.
Washington, D.C. 20055
Call 800-624-6242 or 202-334-3313 (in the Washington metropolitan area)

Printed in the United States of America

The serpent has been a symbol of long life, healing, and knowledge among almost all cultures and religions since the beginning of recorded history. The image adopted as a logotype by the Institute of Medicine is based on a relief carving from ancient Greece, now held by the Staatlichemuseen in Berlin.

COMMITTEE TO REVIEW THE HEALTH CONSEQUENCES OF SERVICE DURING THE PERSIAN GULF WAR

JOHN C. BAILAR III,* *Committee Chair,* Professor and Chair, Department of Health Studies, University of Chicago, Chicago, Illinois

CHRISTOPHER C. GREEN, Executive Director, Research and Development, General Motors Corporation, Warren, Michigan

RICHARD B. HORNICK, Vice-President of Medical Education, Orlando Regional Healthcare System, Medical Education Administration, Orlando, Florida

KARL T. KELSEY, Associate Professor of Occupational Medicine and Radiobiology, Harvard School of Public Health, Boston, Massachusetts

WAYNE M. LEDNAR, Corporate Medical Director, Eastman Kodak Company, Rochester, New York

THOMAS A. LOUIS, Professor and Head, Division of Biostatistics, University of Minnesota School of Public Health, Minneapolis, Minnesota

GARY M. MARSH, Professor, Department of Biostatistics, Graduate School of Public Health, University of Pittsburgh, Pittsburgh, Pennsylvania

DAVID P. RALL,* Institute of Medicine Foreign Secretary, Washington, D.C., Director, Emeritus, National Institute of Environmental Health Sciences, National Institute of Health, Bethesda, Maryland

PHILIP K. RUSSELL, Professor, Department of International Health, School of Hygiene and Public Health, Johns Hopkins University, Baltimore, Maryland

DAVID A. SAVITZ, Professor and Chairman, Department of Epidemiology, School of Public Health, University of North Carolina, Chapel Hill, North Carolina

G. MARIE SWANSON, Director, Cancer Center, and Professor, Department of Family Practice and Medicine, Michigan State University, East Lansing, Michigan

GUTHRIE L. TURNER, Jr., Chief Medical Consultant, Department of Social and Health Services, Division of Disability Determination Services, Washington State, Olympia, Washington

MARK J. UTELL, Professor, Department of Medicine and Environmental Medicine and Director, Pulmonary/Critical Care and Occupational Medicine Divisions, University of Rochester School of Medicine, Rochester, New York

JAMES H. WARE, Dean for Academic Affairs, Harvard School of Public Health, Boston, Massachusetts

DAVID H. WEGMAN, Professor and Chair, Department of Work Environment, University of Massachusetts, Lowell, Massachusetts

---

*Member, Institute of Medicine

LOUIS JOLYON WEST, Professor, Department of Psychiatry and Biobehavioral Sciences, University of California, Los Angeles, School of Medicine, Neuropsychiatric Institute, Los Angeles, California
ELIZABETH A. WILLIAMS, Associate Professor, Department of Internal Medicine, James Quillen College of Medicine, East Tennessee State University, Johnson City, Tennessee
NANCY FUGATE WOODS,* Director, Center for Women's Health Research and Professor, Family and Child Nursing, University of Washington, Seattle, Washington

Study Staff

DIANE J. MUNDT, Study Director
AMANDA H. MURRAY, Research Associate
CARLISS PARKER-SMITH, Project Assistant

Preface

The Committee to Review the Health Consequences of Service During the Persian Gulf War was charged to assess actions taken by the secretaries of the Department of Defense (DoD) and the Department of Veterans Affairs (DVA) to collect and maintain data on the health of Persian Gulf veterans, to make recommendations to improve the collection and maintenance of such data, and to determine whether there is a sound scientific basis for an epidemiologic study of the health consequences of service and, if so, to recommend the types of studies that should be undertaken.

The committee presents 14 findings and 16 recommendations that are intended to improve the nation's understanding of the health consequences of military service in the Persian Gulf, to ameliorate or prevent future health consequences to troops deployed there or in other conflicts, and to improve and accelerate the collection of the information necessary for studying potential problems in the future.

As we publish this report, it will have been about 6 years since approximately 697,000 Americans were deployed to the Persian Gulf, while a nation watched the war unfold on the various news networks. Many questions remain about the health of Persian Gulf veterans and the possible causes of the medical symptoms that many veterans have reported. Some persons believe that a new "Gulf War Syndrome" has appeared and that the symptoms and illnesses that are unexplained are in fact a new disease.

In January 1995, this committee published a first report, *Health Consequences of Service During the Persian Gulf War: Initial Findings and Recommendations for Immediate Action* (Washington, D.C.: National Academy Press), that was critical of the initial actions taken by the DoD and DVA to address these questions, but we are encouraged that these and other organizations have improved their approach to dealing with the medical and social issues in a more organized, coordinated, sympathetic, and effective manner. However, there is still much to do and we trust that the additional recommendations in this report will contribute to further improvements.

The questions of whether a Gulf War veteran is ill and whether that illness was caused by Persian Gulf service are separate and distinct. Our charge and this report address ways to approach the latter question. The former question, although not in the committee's charge, was ever present in its deliberations. The committee was provided with ample evidence that there are veterans who are sick, and we are concerned that they all be provided with proper diagnosis and care.

Those of us who were not in the Gulf can only imagine what it was like for the thousands of men and women who were uprooted from families, jobs, and daily existence; to be suddenly transported to a harsh climate; to be injected with vaccines not previously used in the active military; to wait many months for "action" to occur; to wonder whether the war would involve chemical and biological warfare; to witness a brief but intense battle with many enemy casualties; and then, just as suddenly, to return to their earlier routine of daily living in the United States. Men and women served side by side under conditions that increased the stresses connected with being in these grim surroundings. How all these Gulf experiences relate to the health of veterans is a complex and challenging question.

Although determination of whether a new disease or new syndrome has appeared was not in the committee's charge, we frequently discussed this issue because it helped to enlighten and focus our discussions about the matters we were asked to address. There is a long history in medicine of controversy over the existence of conditions that had not been seen earlier or had not been recognized as separate disease entities. Some of these claimed conditions have faded away, whereas others have become established and generally accepted. Recent examples of the latter are AIDS, Legionnaires' disease, and toxic shock syndrome. For a disease designation to be accepted as valid, criteria need to be set for the diagnosis of that disease so that there will be consistency in reporting. At this time, although studies of Gulf War veterans suggest that these veterans suffer from a variety of recognized diseases, such studies do not establish the existence of a new disease. It is possible that additional findings from research in progress will suggest a new medical entity. Further efforts to identify a Gulf War Syndrome, if it exists, will require substantial new evidence from any research undertaken, but again this issue is separate from whether these ill people need medical care.

Signs and symptoms without a diagnosis or apparent cause are found in every medical practice; clinical medicine is neither perfect nor all-knowing. Although physicians may fail to provide a medical reason for some of these signs and symptoms, the illnesses and related disability have to be addressed as well as possible, independent of efforts to understand causes. All of us in the health care and public health fields are committed to using the scientific study methods available to us in an attempt to understand and better explain what is presently unknown. Only in this way can we make progress in defining, preventing, and treating disease.

Observations, information, and reports by individual veterans provide insight into what it was like to serve in the Gulf, and studies that are now being designed should continue to seek out and consider input from those who were there. Unstructured reports can direct attention to problems that need study, but only rarely can they provide definitive evidence about the appearance of a new medical problem. That is the case with the Gulf War Syndrome. The numerous moving personal stories about illness in returned veterans have rightly generated concern, followed by preliminary research studies. Investigators still will need to use appropriate study designs and methods to obtain the best possible information, conduct equally appropriate analyses, and systematically evaluate the evidence. Knowledge gained in this way will not only benefit the Persian Gulf veterans, but will also help guide DoD and DVA to identify preventive actions that could lessen the likelihood of adverse health outcomes of future deployments. There may also be important extensions to the diagnosis and treatment of exposures and stresses in the civilian population.

Our report is intended to be an evidence-based assessment, so conclusions are inevitably shaped by the evidence that was available at the time the report was written. A substantial research effort is under way, and understanding of the health effects of the Persian Gulf War will evolve as new findings emerge. At the time this report was sent for external review in June 1996, the committee learned that a bunker destroyed in March 1991 may have contained a chemical warfare agent and that troops located 3 or more miles away might have been exposed. DoD officials appearing at a press conference indicated that investigation of this and other incidents is ongoing. Details have since been added (Transcript from President's Advisory Committee on Persian Gulf Veterans' Illnesses, Chicago, Illinois, July 8–9, 1996, and Denver, Colorado, August 6, 1996; Persian Gulf Veterans' Illnesses Investigative Team posting on the Internet, August 6, 1996). The late reporting of this incident and the press conference statement that the investigation of records from the war is still not finished continue to raise questions about the completeness of exposure information provided by DoD to date. We encourage disclosure of all information that may inform the public understanding about the health effects of Persian Gulf service.

As a committee, we are concerned about the health effects of military service, and we are hopeful that DoD and DVA will consider our recommendations to improve the body of information and preventive interventions for the health of Persian Gulf War and future veterans.

Many persons helped the committee in the preparation of this report. First, we have been blessed with an unusually strong staff. Dr. Diane Mundt, as study director, brought to this task a great store of knowledge about epidemiology, biostatistics, military health records, chemical hazards in the field, and related matters, but even more important were her constant oversight of each part of our work and of the role of each committee member; her gently persuasive urging to complete this task, improve on that one, and start a third; and her remarkably comprehensive knowledge about other efforts to understand and improve the health of Gulf War veterans. While the committee wrote the text and takes full responsibility for it, Dr. Mundt's comprehensive attention to improving how we presented our work has made it a far stronger document. Appendixes E, F, and G are among her many contributions. Ms. Amanda Hull Murray was tireless in supporting Dr. Mundt and the committee, with special responsibilities for the critical tasks of learning about and obtaining countless documents (only a fraction could be cited here), coordinating the many presentations to the committee, and aiding veterans and others who had information of potential value to us. Ms. Carliss Parker-Smith supported the work of the office and arranged the details of our 14 committee meetings—no mean task with 18 sometimes fractious committee members and countless other persons simultaneously clamoring for attention to their questions and contributions.

We also thank Ms. Laura Baird and Ms. Susan Fourt for library assistance; Mr. Michael Edington, Ms. Janet Ross, and Ms. Florence Poillon for editorial assistance; many government and nongovernment agencies and organizations for information provided; and countless individuals, including the Persian Gulf veterans who provided both input and insight. Appendixes C and D give some specifics about the persons and organizations who were helpful in this respect.

John C. Bailar III, *Chair*

Contents

APPENDIXES

Executive Summary

On August 2, 1990, a large Iraqi armed force invaded the independent nation of Kuwait. Five days later, U.S. troops began deployment in Operation Desert Shield, and within two months, 200,000 troops had been added to those already in Southwest Asia. By February 1991, more than 500,000 U.S. troops were in the field, facing the Iraqi army. Intense air attacks against the Iraqi armed forces, beginning on January 16, 1991, opened the phase of operations known as Operation Desert Storm (ODS). ODS ended after a brief, but destructive (to the Iraqi forces), ground war from February 24 to February 28, at which time Iraqi resistance was largely ineffective and peace was restored. The number of U.S. troops in the area then declined more rapidly than it had grown. By June 1991, fewer than 50,000 U.S. troops remained. The total number of U.S. military personnel present at one time or another during this interval of Operation Desert Shield/Storm (ODS/S) was about 697,000. The U.S. troops deployed in this war, compared with other conflicts, included a higher proportion of those who were older, were from reserve and guard units, or were female.

The experiences of service personnel were nearly as varied as the individuals deployed, and individuals have responded to their experiences in various ways. The majority of men and women who served in the Gulf returned home and resumed their normal activities with little noticeable difficulty. For others, however, a wide range of physical, chemical, and psychological stressors and exposures appear to have had health effects disproportionate to the brevity of active combat and the relatively low combat casualty rate.

As reports of illnesses and individual complaints increased, so did public concern about a "mystery illness" or "Gulf War Syndrome" (GWS) associated with service in the Persian Gulf (PG). Both the Department of Defense (DoD) and the Department of Veterans Affairs (DVA) were involved from the beginning in tracking and investigating these reports of unexplained signs and symptoms. Efforts in both clinical care and research were initiated, and these have grown in size, complexity, and number.

Speculation about the existence and possible causes of a GWS have involved several federal agencies and numerous research investigators. Many expert opinions have been offered, and a considerable amount of money has been spent. The designation of GWS itself has been controversial. Even without the stress of war, among approximately 697,000 people over a period of several years, there will be poorly understood ailments and a number of obscure diseases.

The work of the committee was determined by its charge, which is derived from Section 706 of Public Law 102-585, in which Congress directed the secretaries of DVA and DoD to seek an agreement with the Medical Follow-up Agency of the Institute of Medicine to review existing scientific, medical, and other information on the health consequences of military service in the PG theater of operations during the Persian Gulf War (PGW).

The committee was charged to assess the effectiveness of actions taken by the secretaries of DVA and DoD to collect and maintain information that is potentially useful for assessing the health consequences of military service referred to in subsection (a) of Public Law 102-585 (PG theater of operations during the PGW); to make recommendations on means of improving the collection and maintenance of such information; and to make recommendations as to whether there is a sound scientific basis for an epidemiologic study or studies of the health consequences of such service and the nature of the study or studies.

To meet this charge, the committee heard presentations and reviewed written materials from representatives of DVA and DoD through May 1996; reviewed relevant scientific literature, protocols, reports of findings, and other documents; held a public meeting; reviewed unsolicited materials received; and attempted through staff updates to keep abreast of relevant PG health-related activities, including activities of other groups.

The committee released a first report in January 1995 with a focus on data and databases, coordination and process, and considerations of study design needs. Little research was under way at that time, and research results were sparse. The first report and this report were written to stand independently, and the recommendations of each are based on the findings and material presented in the individual report.

The committee's charge is specific to DVA and DoD, and the focus of our review of data collection methods and research is specific to those agencies.

Many other activities are being conducted by private individuals, but a comprehensive review of that body of work is beyond the scope of our charge. To make appropriate and relevant recommendations concerning future research activities, the committee believes that a review of federal research activities and plans is appropriate and within the charge. The committee recognizes and agrees that there are veterans who are sick. They must have proper diagnosis and care for their illnesses, including compassionate and expert attention to the full range of their health concerns. However, it is beyond the scope of this committee's work to evaluate issues related to access, responsibility, quality and scope of health care, or possible impact of compensation policies. We believe that this separation of issues is appropriate and that matters of medical care and compensation should be examined separately from issues related to potential causes of illnesses, their treatment, and their prevention in any future conflicts.

Individuals deployed during the PGW were at risk of exposure to a myriad of environmental, occupational, medical, psychological, and battle-related health risks. Some exposures may have occurred in a setting recognized as health threatening; others were unlikely. Some were primarily threats to psychological health; others were threats to physical health. Some potential health effects would be immediate; others would become manifest in the medium term; still others might take years or decades to surface. Within these dimensions, there could be many specific manifestations of symptoms and signs. During and after service in the PGW, veterans did begin to experience adverse health effects. Some of the individuals would have experienced illness during this period whether or not they were in the PGW, whereas the health complaints of others might be a result of their PGW service. However, there is no way to determine which veterans fall into the former group, and research may shed some light on, but not necessarily prove, which may be in the latter group.

Our overarching themes are that reliable and relevant data are essential, that both the broad and the fine details matter a great deal, and that developing an understanding of the range of uncertainty of a risk assessment, while possibly discomforting, may be of greater importance than highlighting best-guess conclusions.

Several good research studies are now under way; attempts are being made to link potential exposures with troop locations; information systems are being improved with regard to data capture (including in-theater tracking), data quality, and intersystem linkages; and the clinical registries of DVA and DoD are obtaining standardized, relevant data.

Even when considering the difficulties and cautions in interpreting research, the committee believes that there is a sound basis for epidemiologic studies, as well as basic science studies, relevant to an understanding of the health consequences of service in the PGW.

There have been special concerns about a range of both naturally occurring and either purposeful or accidental environmental exposures of troops during the

PGW. Objective indicators of harmful environmental exposures in the PG were limited in scope during the PGW and are not readily usable for research purposes. Monitors of air and soil contaminants were not operating for the full period of ODS/S, and other kinds of exposures were not measured. Exposure indicators of other than air or soil were not available. Autopsies of animals and humans, and follow-up examinations of military working dogs, have not indicated the presence of excessive toxic or heavy metals, particularly when data before and after the oil well fires are compared. Official reports of acute health consequences from exposure to air pollutants were rare.

It is clear from written descriptions and reports by veterans that the PG was a hostile environment. Desert conditions, the absence of amenities, uncomfortable temperatures and humidities, extremes in rainfall, blowing sand, insects, animals, fumes, and smoke—all contributed to adverse living conditions. In addition, wartime conditions, including measures uniquely designed to protect the troops, necessitated other exposures such as vaccines against possible biological warfare agents, pyridostigmine bromide to protect against possible chemical warfare agents, and pesticides to protect against bites from insects carrying diseases such as sandfly fever and leishmaniasis. Depleted uranium, used in munitions and tank armor, was a limited but real wartime exposure. Unfortunately, there was no systematic accumulation of data on these exposures, making research into their possible health effects exceptionally difficult, if not impossible.

In the midst of these adverse environmental and wartime-related exposures, soldiers were vulnerable to all of the exposures connected with their particular occupations in the Gulf, such as chemical-agent-resistant coatings, solvents, and vehicle exhaust fumes. Information about "unofficial" exposures, such as the combustion products of leaded fuels in heaters that were sometimes unventilated or nonregulation, wearing flea collars to protect against insect bites, and ingesting alcohol substitutes in the absence of approved alcohol consumption is available only from self-reports.

Not surprisingly, the above scenario creates a picture of an extremely stressful environment, filled with the dangers and trauma of war, combined with a hostile living and work environment. Contributing to this stress were the lack of sanitary conditions and privacy (particularly when men and women were serving together); the speed of being "called-up" to duty and thrown into this environment; "watchful waiting" for the shooting war to begin or SCUD missiles to explode; apprehension heightened by drills and training exercises relating to the threat of chemical and biological warfare; intense workloads; and sleep deprivation. Additionally, issues related to unit cohesion, leadership, morale, and knowledge of family stresses back home varied among individuals but are important for fully understanding the experience of the entire deployed cohort.

Although a wide range of possible exposures might be associated with adverse health outcomes in PG veterans, data on these exposures are often not available; when they are available, they are poorly documented. This lack of exposure information is at the core of the frustration in obtaining answers from epidemiologic studies. Self-reports of exposure and estimation of individual exposures from unit-level measurements will be subject to so much error that they are likely to yield inconclusive results and additional questions.

With the broad question of what adverse health consequences veterans have suffered as a result of their service, the range of relevant experiences is also very broad. The strength of evidence for or against increased risks of specific health outcomes among those who served in the PG depends in part on what research studies have been conducted, and hence, on numerous explicit and implicit decisions made by large numbers of research investigators and funding agencies, often acting individually with little perspective on overall needs and priorities. As a result, the research record is of uneven depth and quality. Our task is to summarize the data available to date that appear relevant to our charge of examining possible health consequences of PGW service and recommend the nature of future studies that would provide more—and better—answers to this question.

Although medical scientists often can use clinical data and individual reports of health experiences to identify areas of concern, such data and reports cannot in themselves provide proof of cause and effect about the health outcomes of PGW service. No matter how well documented an illness may be, or how moving a personal story, unexplained illnesses also occur in the civilian population and in troops not deployed to the Gulf. A basic question regarding the connection between illness in veterans and their service is not whether specific illnesses or adverse health experiences occurred, but whether the frequency or severity of such outcomes was increased over what occurs in otherwise similar populations that were not in the PG.

The range of possible PGW-related health effects that can be studied at this time is intrinsically limited. Illnesses and symptoms that occurred during the deployment and were transient in nature were not studied or monitored systematically then and are very difficult or impossible to study retrospectively now. For example, possible temporary decrements in lung function associated with exposure to pollutants from the oil well fires were not evaluated at the critical time and are not very amenable to study now, although they may be important.

Likewise, health effects that first come to light years after the precipitating exposure cannot easily be studied. Many of the known causes of chronic diseases, such as cancer and coronary artery disease, operate over longer periods than have passed since the PGW and, therefore, cannot yet be evaluated in Gulf War veterans. For example, it is commonly believed that most cancers have a minimum 10-year latent period between exposure and detection of the first extra cases of disease. Thus, although no excess adverse cancer effects have yet been reported, delayed effects that have not yet come to light are still possible. What can be examined now are effects that appear early and are persistent or become manifest at some time up to several years after the relevant exposure.

Concerns about unusual illnesses among PGW veterans arose initially through reports of individuals and then through "outbreak" studies, in which teams of epidemiologists studied groups of soldiers who reported a high prevalence of a cluster of symptoms later proposed to be characteristic of a GWS.

This report reviews three such studies. In each case, the unit came to medical attention because of a report of what appeared to be an unusually high rate of unexplained illness. These studies came to the similar conclusion that troops reported high rates of a variety of nonspecific symptoms, including fatigue, joint pain and stiffness, disturbed or unrefreshing sleep, some gastrointestinal complaints, and a variety of complaints suggestive of mood and musculoskeletal disorders. Thus, although these outbreak studies were successful in demonstrating a common pattern of perceived health problems across a range of military units deployed to the Gulf, they were not successful in demonstrating that these symptoms occurred at a higher rate among PGW veterans than among PG-era veterans (those who did not serve in the PG) or that these symptoms could be linked to specific medical diagnoses or exposures.

To provide some support to those veterans concerned about their health, to enable them to receive a clinical work-up, and to gather information on a possible connection to service in the PG, the DVA and DoD created registries and voluntary referral programs for troops, including DVA's National Referral Center and Persian Gulf Health Registry (PGHR) and DoD's Comprehensive Clinical Evaluation Program (CCEP).

Veterans who have voluntarily participated in these registries have not been found to have any unusual rates of diagnosable conditions but do report a pattern of symptom complaints similar to that seen in the outbreak studies. For example, the five most commonly reported symptoms among registrants in the PGHR were fatigue, headache, skin rash, muscle and joint pain, and loss of memory or other cognitive problems. The registries also share the scientific limitations of the outbreak studies, in that participants are self-selected, symptoms are self-reported, exposures are self-reported and could not be validated, and there is no suitable control group.

Because of these limitations, the committee has concluded that the information on veterans' health that exists in the registries cannot serve alone as a basis for scientific study of the health effects of the PGW. The committee does consider these registries and their affiliated clinical referral programs as useful in assisting veterans who need clinical services and possibly useful as a source of hypotheses regarding the nature and extent of health problems experienced by PGW veterans.

The DVA and various units of the DoD have undertaken a variety of scientific studies of the health status of PGW veterans. The number and scope of these studies have increased rapidly over the past several years, but few studies had been completed as of May 1996. Most of these studies are limited by the absence of detailed exposure information related to individual troops or units. Consequently, studies have had to be designed to seek effects that are sufficiently widespread to be evident when comparing troops who served in the Gulf with those who did not (PG-era veterans).

In seeking evidence for specific effects of service in the PGW, a combination of studies has shown increased rates of symptoms among groups of veterans (many of these being self-selected), with no identified medical diagnosis or exposure. Along with these are studies of mortality and hospitalization rates, in the PG veteran cohort as a whole, that show no consistent differences relative to rates in PG-era veterans. Given this overview, the committee has not identified scientific evidence to date demonstrating adverse health consequences linked with PGW service other than the documented incidents of leishmaniasis, combat-related or injury-related mortality or morbidity, and increased risk of psychiatric sequelae of deployment. At the same time, the committee recognizes that studies provided to us thus far do not comprise a comprehensive scientific investigation of the health consequences of service in the PGW.

The single most troublesome problem encountered in attempts to conduct epidemiologic studies of illnesses among PGW veterans has been the inability to retrieve information on medical care events such as hospitalizations, outpatient visits, and diagnoses and treatments from DoD and DVA medical records in a uniform and systematic manner. Lack of uniform and retrievable medical information concerning reserve, National Guard, active, and separated forces has greatly inhibited systematic analysis of the health effects of mobilization. DoD and DVA have different and only partially automated inpatient hospital record systems. Neither DoD nor DVA has automated outpatient record keeping, although the committee has recently learned that a database with outpatient records will be available in the near future from DVA. Current systems are fragmented, disorganized, incomplete, and therefore poorly suited to support epidemiologic and health outcome studies.

In addition to the PGHR and CCEP mentioned previously, DoD established two other PG database programs: the Troop Exposure Assessment Model (TEAM) and the Registry of Unit Locations (RUL).

The committee finds that the PGHR and CCEP are useful for clinical evaluation of the health problems of PGW veterans but cannot be utilized for research because they include only self-selected individuals who volunteer to participate in these programs. TEAM and RUL also will have limited utility for epidemiologic studies since they provide information at the unit level rather than at the individual level.

Whereas no system of medical record keeping can or should be designed to provide the information needed to address every unanticipated issue regarding the health consequences of either military service in general or a specific military conflict, health information systems can be established to facilitate epidemiologic studies of such service. The committee has identified several changes in health information systems for military personnel that will enhance the capability of the military to evaluate the health consequences of future deployments and service. These changes include creation of a uniform medical record, including data from civilian providers; full implementation of the Defense Medical Epidemiological Database system; and completion of the Army's Patient Accounting and Reporting Real-Time Tracking System (PARRTS), including expansion to the other branches of service.

Medical care and health surveillance (for persons who may need medical attention now) and epidemiologic evaluation of potential threats to the health of service personnel (for research to prevent future problems) will be greatly strengthened by the development of a system that provides access to the entire medical history of each member of the armed services and facilitates linkage to other sources of data. Such a system would provide substantial benefits to the service member and veteran, to future service persons whose health will be better protected, and to DoD or any agency that needs healthy personnel.

As far back as World War I, and perhaps antiquity, every war has left a proportion of service personnel and veterans with serious medical complaints that cannot be explained on the basis of known health hazards or identified physical illnesses. This pattern is so consistent, and the health problems are so important, that databases and health information systems should be designed and implemented now to deal with and mitigate similar problems that are likely to arise in future conflicts.

Two categories of health and exposure information systems are discussed in this report: (1) those established in response to health concerns related to service in the PGW and (2) those developed to improve the future capability to evaluate military-service–related health issues.

Several systems exist for collecting health and exposure information. Some are relevant to clinical evaluations, others are relevant to research, and some are relevant to both. Not all of these information systems are appropriate for use in research activities, nor do they have to be. Some of these systems, such as inpatient hospitalization data, were available at the time of the PGW; others, such as the PGHR, were established shortly thereafter; still others, such as PARRTS, have been developed or extended since the PGW. Some of these systems will be useful for collecting data that strengthen future military health preparedness to address research questions.

The committee considers four steps—(1) the development of a uniform medical record, (2) the improvement of data collection on exposures and health status of deployed service personnel, (3) the provision of supplementary data on occupational and environmental exposures, and (4) the inclusion of early detection medical teams during major deployments—to be important elements of a Military Health Surveillance System that would increase the nation's capacity to address questions about acute and chronic health consequences of deployments of U.S. military service personnel.

In our attempt to investigate comprehensively the health-related consequences of service in the PG, we have encountered numerous hypotheses, often provided by independent investigators, that have suggested a wide variety of associations among agents and exposures, circumstances that existed in the Gulf, and adverse clinical outcomes. These hypotheses have had varying degrees of plausibility and supporting research. Some investigators brought their work to the attention of the committee. In each case, the material presented by individuals and groups, in person or in documents, was evaluated by the entire committee and considered as we formed our overall impression of the health consequences of service in the Gulf. The many investigations (both federal and private) and the putative causal associations that we evaluated demonstrate the vexing nature of the medical problem presented by what some have referred to as a Gulf War Syndrome, and we refer to here as unexplained illnesses (UI).

A précis of many of the hypotheses and much of the supporting evidence that the committee received is provided in the report. Most of this material was not solicited. Thus, this list is not intended to be exhaustive or complete but rather to illustrate the issues that faced both the investigators and the committee. The number and variety of hypotheses call attention to the variety of different types of abnormalities that have been reported and the strong likelihood that no single hypothesis could account for all of these, whether or not the illnesses result from service in the PGW.

The committee has been troubled by news stories about activities to promote the treatment of clinically evident manifestations of UI. These raise ethically troublesome questions about the lack of documented efficacy, and some of these interventions could even prove harmful to individual patients. Since placebo treatment of patients with almost any ailment (psychological or otherwise) will often result in marked improvement in symptoms or even physical signs of disease, well-designed clinical studies must be employed to understand the efficacy of any medical intervention.

Finally, although the committee has not identified an explanation for the unexplained illnesses in PG veterans, we do not doubt that many individuals reporting such illness are seriously affected. We recognize that many illnesses in the population at large lack explanation according to current medical understanding and also require an open mind. Continuing efforts to explore all possible avenues to increase our knowledge of such illnesses, and to reduce suffering and disability, are certainly indicated. The fact that work of the tentative nature summarized in the report continues 6 years after cessation of the

PGW underscores the importance of taking seriously the reports of ill health among active and returning troops. Those involved in future conflicts must anticipate the need to integrate into DoD and DVA planning at all stages high-quality research on the health consequences of combat and of deployments to hostile environments.

The committee makes recommendations in this report regarding the collection and maintenance of information that is potentially useful for assessing the health consequences of military service in the PGW. These recommendations support completion of certain data sets, prompt reporting of research findings and submission for publication in peer-reviewed journals, strengthened medical and epidemiologic research capabilities of the armed forces, and strengthening the decision-making processes for study selection.

We also give considerable attention to information systems that would be useful in future conflicts. These recommendations are based largely on experience with systems in place for the PGW that have shown some gaps and defects that can be remedied.

The committee believes that there is indeed a sound basis for epidemiologic studies, and recommendations follow. However, the committee does not recommend an additional nationwide epidemiologic study of PG veterans, because such a study is likely to be of limited scientific value at this time. Those large studies that are currently under way should be completed as quickly as possible, while continuing to meet high scientific standards, including a high response rate and a thorough investigation of potential biases, as recommended below.

The recommendations are listed here without their associated findings. The reader is referred to the full report for the associated and specific findings supporting each recommendation.

RECOMMENDATIONS

Recommendation 1. The DoD, the branches of the armed services, and the DVA should continue to work together to develop, fund, and staff medical information systems that include a single, uniform, continuous, and retrievable electronic medical record for each service person. The uniform record should include each relevant health item (including baseline personal risk factors, every inpatient and outpatient medical contact, and all health-related interventions), allow linkage to exposure and other data sets, and have the capability to incorporate relevant medical data from beyond the DoD and DVA institutions (e.g., U.S. Public Health Service facilities, civilian medical providers, and other health care institutions). Appropriate consent and protection of individual privacy must be considered for information obtained and included.

Recommendation 2. The DoD and DVA should conduct further studies, with appropriate statistical and epidemiological support, to identify risk factors for stress-related psychiatric disorders among military personnel (active and reserve) and to develop better methods to buffer and ameliorate the psychiatric consequences of modern training, deployment, combat, demobilization, and return to daily living.

Recommendation 3. Studies being conducted by DoD and DVA that have included longitudinal follow-up of the mental health of veterans who served in the PG should be supported with continued follow-up, after appropriate peer review of study methods. Follow-up in these studies should be sufficient to provide at least a decade of information comparing the mental health status of those deployed with those not deployed.

Recommendation 4. The DoD should ensure that military medical preparedness for deployments includes detailed attempts to monitor natural and man-made environmental exposures and to prepare for rapid response, early investigation, and accurate data collection, when possible, on physical and natural environmental exposures that are known or possible in the specific theater of operations.

Recommendation 5. Research is needed to determine whether differences in personal characteristics or differences in policies and procedures for mobilization, deployment, demobilization, and return of reserves, National Guard, and regular troops are associated with different or adverse health consequences. If there are associations, strategies necessary to prevent or reduce these adverse health effects should be developed.

Recommendation 6. The mortality experience of PG veterans should continue to be monitored for as long as 30 years, on a regular basis, including comparisons with that of PG-era veterans. (PG-era veterans have been defined as those in military service at the time of the PGW, but assigned or deployed elsewhere.) Research investigators should focus on the reported excess mortality from unintentional injury, on mortality from specific illnesses, and on evidence of elevation (or reduction) in the risk of death from other causes.

Recommendation 7. The DVA should exert greater effort to improve understanding of the reasons for excess mortality from unintentional injury. Detailed evaluation is needed beyond death certificate data concerning the circumstances surrounding fatal injury, through more focused case-control studies to identify both individual risk factors and remediable causes.

Recommendation 8. The Defense Medical Epidemiological Database system should be continued, expanded as planned, expedited to develop the proposed integrated information management system, linked to other key systems, and evaluated regularly.

Recommendation 9. The DoD should complete development of information systems to expeditiously and directly pinpoint unit locations at a high level of disaggregation in space and time (that is, fine detail) and to document local environmental conditions, including appropriate data quality checks, with direct data entry into the system. There is likely to be a need for a similar information system during and after any future conflict, and DoD should prepare and continually update plans for such a nonpaper system. A manual for use of the information systems by research investigators should be compiled, with the strengths and limitations identified.

Recommendation 10. For every specific question posed to the current TEAM, DoD should assess the strengths and limitations of the TEAM as a resource for evaluating the health significance of geographically defined exposures of troops, including those in the PGW and those in conflicts that may develop in the future. Evaluations and recommendations for possible modification of the TEAM should be reported to the PG Coordinating Board, Research Working Group.

Recommendation 11. The DoD and DVA should ensure that studies of the health effects of deployment, including effects on PGW veterans, include evaluation of the exposures, experiences, and situations of both women and men, with attention to their age, prior military service, marital and parental status, and other gender-specific parameters.

Recommendation 12. The DoD and DVA should conduct studies of the health consequences of assigning men and women to serve together in combat or under the threat of enemy action. Such work should be undertaken with a focus on prevention and amelioration of any added stresses.

Recommendation 13a. The Naval Health Research studies in San Diego should be completed and results published as designed and scheduled.

Recommendation 13b. The DVA National Health Survey should be completed and results published as designed and scheduled.

Recommendation 13c. Evaluation of predictors of enrollment in the DVA PGHR should be promptly completed and results published. Included, if possible, should be information on type of care requested, required, and received.

Recommendation 14. The epidemiologic capabilities of the armed forces should be strengthened rather than reduced. The command structure should be kept informed about the reasons for and the results of this recommendation and its relevance to military preparedness and effectiveness, and should be encouraged to support appropriate epidemiologic work in the theater of operations and in the postdeployment period.

Recommendation 15. The DoD and DVA should adopt a policy that internal and contract-supported reports on health research will be submitted for publication in the peer-reviewed scientific literature in a timely manner.

Recommendation 16. The Congress, DVA, and DoD should adopt a policy that unless there are well-specified, openly stated reasons to the contrary, requests for proposals for research related to unexplained illnesses or other needed health-related research will be publicly announced and open to the scientific community at large, that proposals will be reviewed by panels of appropriately qualified experts, and that funding will follow the recommendations of those experts.

1

Introduction

On August 2, 1990, a large Iraqi armed force invaded the independent nation of Kuwait. Five days later, U.S. troops began deployment in Operation Desert Shield, and within 2 months, 200,000 troops had been added to those already in Southwest Asia (SWA). By February 1991, more than 500,000 U.S. troops were in the field, facing the Iraqi army. Intense air attacks against the Iraqi armed forces, beginning on January 16, 1991, opened the phase of operations known as Operation Desert Storm (ODS). ODS ended after a brief, but destructive (to the Iraqi forces), ground war from February 24 to February 28, at which time Iraqi resistance was largely ineffective and peace was restored. The number of U.S. troops in the area then declined more rapidly than it had grown. By June 1991, fewer than 50,000 U.S. troops remained. The total number of U.S. military personnel present at one or another time during this interval of Operation Desert Shield/Desert Storm (ODS/S) was about 697,000. The U.S. troops deployed in this war, compared with other conflicts, included a higher proportion of those who were older, were from reserve and guard units, or were female.

Although the ground war was short, U.S. service persons experienced several kinds of major, sometimes quite unusual stresses in addition to limited combat. Some of these were physiological, but many were from recognized environmental and external agents such as diesel fumes; microbes; the hostile, hot sandy desert environment; vaccines; oil well fires; and specific occupational exposures. However, there were also potent psychological stresses of several kinds. One was the sudden disruption of lives of large numbers of persons, including family strains when military reserves were suddenly called to active duty. A second was the unfamiliar character of the region and the requirement that U.S. military personnel have virtually no interaction with the indigenous populations. A third was the very primitive conditions into which some troops were placed. Such basic matters as permanent structures for living or even tents, frequent hot meals, laundry, and recreation were not widely available until near the peak of the military buildup. Other stresses on service personnel came from personal reactions to the very success of the brief war, including the immense destruction visited on the whole nation of Iraq. An additional stressor, unique to this war, was the virtually immediate news reporting of the progress of the war and the ability of those at home to share the images and resulting concerns. This new level of detail in reporting and immediacy of communication intensified the impact of the war experience for those in the field. The dangers from Soviet-designed surface-to-surface (SCUD) missiles were well known. In addition, reports, training, and widespread news related to the "virtual certainty" that chemical and biological warfare (CBW) agents would be used by Iraq in the Gulf theater served to raise levels of apprehension.

The experiences of service personnel were nearly as varied as the individuals deployed, and individuals have responded to their experiences in different ways. The majority of men and women who served in the Gulf returned home and resumed their normal activities with little noticeable difficulty. For others, however, a wide range of physical, chemical, and psychological stressors and exposures appear to have had health effects disproportionate to the brevity of active combat and the relatively low combat casualty rate.

AN EMERGING PROBLEM

In April 1991, while troops were still returning home from the Gulf, Congress passed legislation (Public Law [PL] 102-25) requiring the Secretary of Defense and the Secretary of Veterans Affairs to assess the need for rehabilitative services for those participating in Operation Desert Storm who experienced posttraumatic stress disorder (PTSD); to describe available programs and resources to meet those needs; to describe specific plans for treatment of members experiencing PTSD, particularly with respect to any special needs of members of reserve components; and to provide an assessment of needs for additional resources necessary to carry out such plans, with a description of plans for each department (Department of Defense [DoD] and Department of Veterans Affairs [DVA]) to coordinate treatment services for PTSD with the other. This early action resulted in several DVA projects that are cited in Appendix F of this report.

There were also general concerns about possible health effects of exposure to the oil well fires, and as early as April 1991, DVA developed a Persian Gulf Health Registry (PGHR) examination to provide a clinical work-up for veterans concerned about possible Persian Gulf (PG) service-related illnesses. The DVA registry was later mandated in PL 102-585 (Appendix A) as the DVA Persian Gulf War Veterans Health Registry, to include all who served in the Gulf (whether their present status was active, reserve, or National Guard, including those who left the service). This law (PL 102-585) also expanded previous legislation (PL 102-90, December 1991) mandating that the DoD registry of troops exposed to burning oil well fires include not only those exposed to fires but also all who served in the SWA theater of operations during the Persian Gulf War (PGW).

However, the registries were not designed to answer questions about health complaints such as those that soon started to emerge from some veterans who had served in the PGW.[1] In January 1992, there were reports from the 123rd Army Reserve Unit in Indiana of unexpected signs and symptoms that could not easily be explained.[2] This cluster of reports was investigated by researchers from the Walter Reed Army Institute of Research (WRAIR), who found no common exposures among these reserve troops that could account for the signs and symptoms reported (DeFraites et al., 1992). This "outbreak" was reported in the news media and received considerable attention. Veterans in other units also began to report their own signs and symptoms, often including serious fatigue, joint pains, headaches, and sleep complaints.

As reports of such illnesses and individual complaints increased, so did public concern about a "mystery illness" or "Gulf War Syndrome" (GWS) associated with service in the PG. Both DoD and DVA were involved from the beginning in tracking and investigating these reports of unexplained signs and symptoms. Efforts in both clinical care and research were initiated, and these have grown in size, complexity, and number.

The DVA's PGHR was initially associated with three referral centers (Washington, D.C.; Houston, Texas; and West Los Angeles, California) that moved toward standardized and extensive protocols and procedures in 1994. Beginning in June 1994, DoD started a clinical evaluation (Comprehensive Clinical Evaluation Program [CCEP]) specific to active duty troops and modeled after DVA's referral center examinations. An additional referral center in Birmingham, Alabama, was added by DVA in 1995. Research and clinical activities related to a possible GWS and to other health consequences of service in the PGW have multiplied to the point that it is now becoming difficult to keep track of all of the research programs, clinical evaluations, and special treatment efforts.

---

[1]We sometimes use the term "veteran" for those who served in the PG but may still be on duty elsewhere; sometimes the term refers to those who have left military service.

[2]We generally use "symptoms" to refer to subjective experiences (such as pain or fatigue) described by patients and "signs" to refer to objective findings (such as reduced lung capacity or abnormal reflexes) that a trained observer can detect, perhaps with help from the laboratory.

Speculation about the existence and possible causes of a GWS have involved several federal agencies and numerous research investigators. Many expert opinions have been offered, and a considerable amount of money has been spent. The designation of GWS itself has been controversial. Even without the stress of war, among approximately 697,000 people over a period of several years, there will be poorly understood ailments and a number of obscure diseases.

Beyond these, stress alone can lead to serious illness and disability, often chronic. For example, in comparing long-term outcomes in Japanese atomic bomb survivors with those in Japanese persons who were not exposed, Schull (1996) recently noted that "these studies have shown that as a group the survivors have anxieties not shared with Japanese who were not exposed. They often complain of what has been termed *hibakusha, bura-bura*—the occurrence of lingering fatigue and medically ill-defined symptoms for which no biological basis could be found."

PANELS AND COMMITTEES

As initial actions described in the previous section were being undertaken by DoD and DVA, White House and congressional interest and involvement also grew rapidly. A number of committees or special groups were established to inspect, review, or evaluate various aspects of the PG veterans health issue (Appendix E). One of the first of these committees met in May 1993. In response to a growing concern that PG veterans were experiencing unexplained illnesses, DVA held a meeting of an informal "blue-ribbon panel" of experts. The group was subsequently chartered (October 8, 1993) as the PG Expert Scientific Committee to advise the DVA Assistant Chief Medical Director for Environmental Medicine and Public Health, and subsequently the DVA Undersecretary for Health, about medical findings affecting PG veterans. The committee was charged to review all aspects of patient care and medical diagnoses and to provide professional consultation as needed. The DVA committee could advise on other areas involving research and development, veterans benefits, and training for patients and staff. The newly chartered committee, chaired by Dr. Eula Bingham, University of Cincinnati, first met in February 1994, approximately once per quarter through 1995, and once in 1996.

Previously mentioned legislation (PL 102-585) also directed DVA and DoD to seek an agreement with the Medical Follow-up Agency (MFUA) of the Institute of Medicine (IOM), one of three major components of the National Academy of Sciences (NAS), to review the collection and maintenance of data on health consequences of the PGW, consider reported health outcomes, and recommend appropriate studies.

Experts in biostatistics, epidemiology, general medicine, infectious diseases, neurotoxicology, nutrition, psychiatry, pulmonary health, reproductive health, toxicology, vaccines, and women's health issues were assembled. The work of the committee began when it was funded on October 1, 1993. The committee first met on January 20–21, 1994, and held a total of 14 meetings during the two and a half years it was active (Appendix C). A first report, focused primarily on the research process rather than findings, was released on January 4, 1995 (IOM, 1995a). This second and final report of the committee includes information received and evaluated through May 1996.

Also, at the end of 1993, DoD assembled a group of experts to examine reports of illnesses that could not be diagnosed. As requested by the Undersecretary of Defense in December 1993, a task force of the DoD Defense Science Board (DSB) was charged to review scientific and medical evidence relating to long-term health effects of exposure to low levels of neurotoxic agents. The Defense Science Board's Task Force on Persian Gulf War Health Effects first met in December 1993. Dr. Joshua Lederberg of Rockefeller University chaired the proceedings. After the first meeting, the task force requested that the charge be changed to focus deliberations on the cause and effect of the full range of exposures to low levels of chemicals as well as environmental pollutants, endemic biologics, and other health hazards that might affect veterans of the PGW. An interim report was released on March 15, 1994; the final report was released in June 1994 (DSB, 1994). The medical nature and the cause or causes of a GWS remained undefined by the task force. The DSB task force did not find evidence of any specific cause-effect relation between putative exposures and an undefined illness. Furthermore, the DSB task force was convinced that reported illnesses by PGW veterans were not due to chemical or biological warfare agents.

On August 31, 1993, President Clinton designated DVA as the lead agency to coordinate all research activities undertaken or funded by the executive branch on the health consequences of military service in the PG theater of operations during the PGW. This coordination, mandated by PL 102-585, includes the DVA, DoD, Department of Health and Human Services (DHHS), and Environmental Protection Agency (EPA).

As concern about unexplained illness among PG veterans continued to grow, on January 1994 the secretaries of Defense, Veterans Affairs, and Health and Human Services formed a Persian Gulf Veterans Coordinating Board (PGVCB) to ensure interagency coordination of all efforts—both separate and joint—in research, clinical care, and disability determination and compensation for illnesses after ODS/S; to ensure effective and broad application of resources; and to provide means of disseminating information. The research coordination occurs under the activities of the Research Working Group (RWG) of the PGVCB, charged with "assessing the state and direction of research; identifying gaps in factual knowledge and conceptual understanding; identifying testable hypotheses; recommending research directions for participating agencies; reviewing research concepts as they are developed; and collecting and disseminating scientifically peer-reviewed information" (PGVCB, 1995b).

One of the first activities sponsored jointly by the RWG and the National Institutes of Health (NIH) was a Technology Assessment Workshop held April 27–29, 1994, "The Persian Gulf Experience and Health" (NIH Technology Assessment Workshop Panel, 1994). This two-and-a-half-day workshop considered four questions: (1) What is the evidence for an increased incidence of unexpected illnesses attributable to service in the PGW? (2) If unexpected illnesses have occurred, what are the components of the most practical working case definition(s) based on existing data? (3) If unexpected illnesses have occurred, what are the plausible etiologies and biological explanations for these unexpected illnesses? (4) What future research is necessary?

The panel was unable to develop a definition of GWS that could be used to determine whether there is an association between exposures (plausible etiologies) and outcomes (otherwise unexplained illnesses). It criticized the lack of research and available data and focused its recommendations on (1) a short health questionnaire aimed at all 697,000 people who served in the PGW, (2) a focused hospital–clinical protocol for DoD and DVA to use in their research on chronic fatigue syndrome, (3) designs for cohort and case-control studies of health effects of the PGW, (4) a retrospective cohort study of pulmonary function in veterans, (5) retrospective simulation of exposures of possible health interest, (6) research into potential stressors, (7) development of effective responses to diagnosis and treatment of stress-related conditions, (8) planning for prospective data collection, and (9) further research on leishmaniasis, which had been suggested as a possible cause of illness in PG veterans (NIH Technology Assessment Workshop Panel, 1994).

Our first report criticized the agencies for their lack of coordination (IOM, 1995a). We believe that, since that time, the RWG has made considerable progress in developing a unified federal research plan to examine PG health issues. The group released *A Working Plan for Research on Persian Gulf Veterans' Illnesses* in August 1995 (PGVCB, 1995b), which, although "intended to guide federal decision makers in establishing research spending priorities, it is also meant to provide information to members of Congress, the scientific community, the public, and, most importantly, the veterans of the Persian Gulf conflict, about the manner in which the federal government is carrying out the research mandate." This document was scheduled to be updated in the spring of 1996 but was not available for review by this IOM committee. The first version of the RWG working plan was an attempt to put the various research activities currently under way into a structure that reflected possible hypotheses as well as gaps in current research.

An earlier version of the RWG working plan had been made available to researchers who were interested in responding to a DoD Broad Area

Announcement (BAA) requesting proposals for research in three areas mandated by Congress in PL 103-337: epidemiology, effects of pyridostigmine bromide (PB), and clinical research. The three BAAs were announced in May 1995 and generated more than 100 responses, which were reviewed for scientific merit by scientists selected by the American Institute of Biological Sciences (AIBS). These reviews, with respondent's name and affiliation removed, were submitted to the RWG for ranking within areas mandated by law and priorities for PG research as set forth in the working plan. Although recommendations were made in January 1996 by the RWG as to the top 12 proposals to be funded, as of the end of May 1996, the announcements of awards had not been made. Therefore, this committee cannot comment on the scope and quality of work selected, which includes three epidemiologic studies, two studies of the effects of PB, five clinical studies, one environmental study, and one leishmania study (Mather, 1996).

The most recently established official group to review the health concerns of PG veterans is the Presidential Advisory Committee (PAC) on Gulf War Veterans' Illnesses, established by Executive Order 12961, May 26, 1995. The PAC was charged to review research, coordinating efforts, medical treatment, outreach, external reviews, risk factors, and chemical and biological weapons. As of May 1996, PAC had held six full committee meetings and five panel meetings. Speakers invited by PAC have testified on specific topics on which information has been requested. All meetings have included an opportunity for public comment. Meetings have been held across the United States to allow greater participation by PG veterans. An interim report, issued in February 1996 (PAC, 1996a), focused on outreach, medical and clinical issues, research, and chemical and biological weapons. The final PAC report is expected in December 1996.

CONCLUSIONS

Deliberations of these committees and panels have contributed to public interest in the health concerns of PG veterans. Considerable constituent pressure on members of Congress has resulted in legislation mandating agencies to appropriate funds for individual research projects and legislation mandating broad classes of studies, as described above. The committee stresses that for some of the studies designated in this manner, the quality of the individual study is not the issue, but whether the right studies have been selected for support. Such selection requires considerable technical judgment to ensure that the most relevant populations are examined, that the research has the maximum power to detect effects, and that the cost–benefit ratio is the best that can be attained.

We are concerned by the appropriation of funds for individual scientists who have not had peer-reviewed research protocols or whose protocols have not passed funding agency scientific and institutional review boards. Failure to adhere to accepted standards and sidestepping of the peer-reviewed research process can result in inferior, worthless, or even unethical research, leading to the adoption of diagnoses and treatments that are medically and ethically questionable and possibly harmful.

CHARGE TO THE COMMITTEE

The work of the committee was determined by its charge, which is derived from Section 706 of PL 102-585, in which Congress directed the secretaries of DVA and DoD to seek an agreement with the MFUA of the IOM to review existing scientific, medical, and other information on the health consequences of military service in the PG theater of operations during the PGW (see Appendix A). The committee's Statement of Task (Appendix B) was drafted by IOM, DVA, and DoD in response to that legislation. A letter from Representative Sonny Montgomery (Former Chairman, House Committee on Veterans Affairs) and Senator John D. Rockefeller IV (Former Chairman, Senate Committee on Veterans Affairs), received shortly after the committee's first meeting, asked for a broader interpretation of the work of the committee than was in the original charge. The committee has responded to this request by discussing and making recommendations within the context of the charge on issues that may impact the health and related matters of soldiers in future deployments.

To meet this charge, the committee heard presentations (Appendix D) and reviewed written materials from representatives of DVA and DoD through May 1996; reviewed relevant scientific literature, protocols, reports of findings, and other documents; held a public meeting; reviewed unsolicited materials received (Appendix C); and attempted through staff updates to keep abreast of relevant PG health-related activities, including the activities of other groups.

The committee released a first report in January 1995 with a focus on data and databases, coordination and process, and considerations of study design needs. Little research was under way at that time, and research results were sparse. The first report and this report were written to stand independently, and the recommendations of each are based on the findings and material presented in the individual report.

The first report of this committee was critical of the lack of research coordination. This lack appears to have been largely repaired by the activities of the RWG of the PGVCB, to the extent that this committee was able to observe their actions. However, it is difficult for outsiders to make specific and appropriate recommendations on how the DoD and DVA should coordinate future research efforts (as distinct from how to conduct specific research programs and projects), because the two agencies are so different, including differences in their areas of research strength. Although issues of how research on health outcomes from future conflicts should be coordinated were beyond the scope of this committee's charge, we believe that it is extremely important for DVA and DoD to find strategic solutions to problems of joint research efforts.

The committee's charge is specific to DVA and DoD, and the focus of our review of data collection methods and research is specific to those agencies. Terminology used in the report necessarily reflects that used by these sponsors. Many other activities are being conducted by private individuals, but a comprehensive review of that body of work is beyond the scope of our charge. However, to make appropriate and relevant recommendations concerning future research activities, the committee believes that a review of federal research activities and plans is appropriate and within the charge. The committee recognizes and agrees that there are veterans who are sick. They must have proper diagnosis and care for their illnesses, including compassionate and expert attention to the full range of their health concerns. However, it is beyond the scope of this committee's work to evaluate issues related to access, responsibility, quality and scope of health care, or possible impact of compensation policies. We believe that this separation of issues is appropriate and that matters of medical care and compensation should be examined separately from issues related to potential causes of illnesses, their treatment, and their prevention in any future conflicts.

RESEARCH AND DATA ISSUES

Because the task before this committee is focused so heavily on research and data collection efforts, we discuss herein some issues of research design that will provide a framework for the more detailed comments in subsequent chapters. More extensive discussions of epidemiologic research design and definitions of epidemiologic terms can be found in standard references (Fletcher et al., 1995; Lillienfeld and Stolley, 1994).

As we have indicated, individuals deployed during the PGW were at risk of exposure to a myriad of environmental, occupational, medical, psychological, and battle-related health risks. Some exposures may have occurred in a setting recognized as health threatening; other exposures were unlikely. Some were primarily threats to psychological health; others were threats to physical health. Some potential health effects would be immediate; others would become manifest in the medium term; still others might take years or decades to surface. Within these dimensions, there could be many specific manifestations of symptoms and signs. During and after service in the PGW, veterans did begin to experience adverse health effects. Some were PGW-related. Other individuals would have experienced illness during this period whether or not they were in the PGW, whereas the health complaints of still others might be a result of their PGW service. However, there is no way to determine which veterans fall into the former group, and research may shed some light on, but not necessarily prove, which may be in the latter group.

The most important clinical goal is to understand and treat individual illness. This is complementary to, but distinct from, scientific and public health goals and should be pursued as appropriate without regard to causes or mechanisms of disease. The scientific and public health goals will require relating various exposures and environments to health outcomes. A better understanding of this relation will of course help in attaining the clinical goal. Achievement of the scientific and public health goals might benefit PGW veterans but also allows for prevention or amelioration of adverse health outcomes for troops deployed in the future and for the general population. However, success in attaining the scientific and public health goals will require reliable and relevant information, scientifically sound analysis and interpretation, and availability of effective treatment and prevention resources and modalities.

To provide a framework for our recommendations in Chapter 2 and for the evaluations in subsequent chapters, we outline some key scientific and procedural issues related to health risk assessment goals. Our overarching themes are that reliable and relevant data are essential, that both broad and fine details matter a great deal, and that developing an understanding of the range of uncertainty of a risk assessment, while possibly discomforting, may be of greater importance than highlighting best-guess conclusions.

The ultimate goal of a health risk assessment is to help in the control of risk by identifying and quantifying its determinants, understanding differences in susceptibility, and assessing levels of exposure (NRC, 1983, 1993). Some risk factors may be modifiable (e.g., environmental exposures or quality of troop leadership), whereas knowledge of others may be useful in tactical planning (e.g., certain individuals should not be exposed to certain noxious agents). Features of the PGW context as a less than ideal research setting are discussed. These lead to our recommendations in the following chapter and the detailed analysis in subsequent chapters.

The PGW as the Less-than-Ideal Setting for Research

No health risk assessment is ever undertaken in a fully idealized setting, and our evaluations of the PGW situation should be taken in this context and in recognition of the limitations inherent in any health risk assessment. Conditions and situations in the Gulf theater were not conducive for the proper conduct of research on health outcomes. Some of the problems encountered could be eliminated or ameliorated (databases can be, and are being, improved); for others, progress will be difficult (personal exposures in the theater of operations were not measured and cannot be reconstructed); still others are the inevitable consequence of the early phases of any scientific investigation (no agreed disease definition, poorly formulated or nonexistent hypotheses leading to poorly collected data, or the absence of data on potentially important inputs and outputs).

As the committee noted in its first report (IOM, 1995a), initial research efforts were poorly organized both strategically (what studies could and should be conducted) and tactically (how they should be conducted). For many data collection and analysis activities, no reference population was available (e.g., the registries or outbreak studies), predeployment demographic information on health and medical interventions such as vaccinations was incomplete and possibly inaccurate, there was little standardization and operationalization of data on disease symptoms and signs, follow-up was difficult and incomplete (DoD and DVA databases did not communicate effectively), very little personalized exposure information was available, and changes over time made some data unavailable and reduced or modified possible reference populations. Defining relevant control groups and obtaining data for them were very difficult. The full range of potential biases (selection bias, follow-up bias, dropout bias, observation bias, ascertainment bias, and recall bias) was operating. These problems further limit the ability of even the most expert and well-funded investigation to identify health outcomes linked to specific exposures or risk factors. These and other issues are discussed in detail in subsequent chapters. One example of the challenges posed by the PGW situation is associated with cluster identification.

There are specific problems associated with studies of "clusters" of some illnesses (Rothman, 1990) (also called outbreak studies or "hot pursuit" studies, characterized as fast, preliminary investigations). Even if the disease is well defined and its diagnosis is properly operationalized, clusters cannot be used to evaluate causation because it is virtually impossible to identify a reference population. Clusters will arise in the absence of causation; indeed they are inevitable in any large and complex collection of study participants and data. It is the task of the investigating analyst to sort out clusters that occur by chance from those that occur as a result of some exposure of interest.

Clusters sometimes arise, are publicized, generate interest, and often lead to the collection of "cases" (numerator data) that are poorly defined with little knowledge of populations at risk (denominator data). Clusters can play an important role in helping to formulate hypotheses for subsequent studies, and initial reports from sick PG veterans were the starting point for certain types of questions asked in early PG research surveys—for example, prevalence of fatigue, headache, muscle aches, and weakness. However, neither well-documented clusters nor moving stories of personal tragedy ("clusters" of one) can establish a cause–effect link between some experience or exposure and a health outcome.

Where Do We Go from Here?

The foregoing paints a rather bleak portrait of the PGW context for health risk assessment. This pessimism is in some ways warranted, but several positive developments could help in evaluating the PGW deployment and any future deployments. Several good research studies are now under way; attempts are being made to link potential exposures with troop locations; information systems are being improved with regard to data capture (including in-theater tracking), data quality, and intersystem linkages; and the clinical registries of DVA and DoD are obtaining standardized, relevant data.

Even when considering the difficulties and cautions in interpreting research as described above, the committee believes that there is a sound basis for epidemiologic studies, as well as basic science studies, relevant to an understanding of health consequences of service in the PGW. Specific recommendations about the nature of those studies are presented in Chapter 2. A list of acronyms is provided to assist the reader. Each chapter begins with an "Overview" that summarizes the major points in that chapter.

2

Charge to the Committee: Its Findings and Recommendations

OVERVIEW

In this chapter we summarize the findings and principal recommendations of the Committee to Review the Health Consequences of Service During the Persian Gulf War (PGW). Most of the findings are discussed at greater length in the chapters that follow.

Our task was to respond to three specific charges. Each finding is linked to at least one of the charges, and for each we note the principal connection. Recommendations follow each of the findings. The committee was charged as follows:

THE COMMITTEE'S CHARGE

Charge 1

> Assess the effectiveness of actions taken by the Secretary of Veterans Affairs and the Secretary of Defense to collect and maintain information that is potentially useful for assessing the health consequences of military service referred to subsection (a) [of PL 102-585, Persian Gulf (PG) theater of operations during the PGW].

The committee makes four recommendations (recommendations 13–16) in this report regarding the collection and maintenance of information that is potentially useful for assessing the health consequences of military service in the PGW. These recommendations support completion of certain data sets, prompt reporting of research findings and submission for publication in peer-reviewed journals, strengthened medical and epidemiologic research capabilities of the armed forces, and strengthening the decision-making processes for study selection.

Charge 2

> Make recommendations on means of improving the collection and maintenance of such information.

The committee makes five recommendations (recommendations 1, 4, and 8–10) on the collection and maintenance of information on the health consequences of service in the PG. We also give considerable attention to information systems that would be useful in future conflicts. These recommendations are based largely on experience with systems in place for the PGW that have shown some gaps and defects that can be remedied.

Charge 3

> Make recommendations as to whether there is [a] sound scientific basis for an epidemiologic study or studies of the health consequences of such service, and if the recommendation is that there is [a] sound scientific basis for such a study or studies, the nature of the study or studies.

The committee believes that there is indeed a sound basis for epidemiologic studies, and eight recommendations follow (recommendations 2, 3, 5–7, and 11–13).[1] However, the committee does not recommend an additional nationwide epidemiologic study of PG veterans, because such a study is likely to be of limited scientific value at this time. Those large studies that are currently under way should be completed as quickly as possible, while meeting high scientific standards, including a high response rate and a thorough investigation of potential biases, as recommended below.

---

[1] Recommendation 13 has been counted as applicable to both Charge 1 and Charge 3, and therefore appears with both.

FINDINGS AND RECOMMENDATIONS

Finding

Recent military deployments, especially in Vietnam and in the Persian Gulf, have demonstrated that concerns about the health consequences of participation in military action may arise long after deployment has ended and that the evaluation of those concerns and the provision of health care to affected personnel may present formidable challenges both to epidemiologists and to medical caregivers. Although some of these challenges can be attributed to the intrinsic difficulty of evaluating poorly understood clusters of events that were not among the expected consequences of combat or of environmental conditions, they also may be attributed in part to limitations of the systems used to collect and manage data regarding the health and service-related exposures of military personnel. No system of record keeping can be expected to provide the information needed to address every unanticipated research issue, including those regarding the health consequences of military service. Nevertheless, the committee has identified several possible improvements in the systems and practices for collecting information on the health and service-related exposures of military personnel. Such changes would increase the ability of the military services to pursue appropriate investigations in the future. Such changes also would increase the capacity of the services to evaluate the efficacy of mobilization-supporting health services (including approaches and methodologies for disease prevention employed before, during, and after mobilization) and would aid in providing the best possible medical care to military service personnel and veterans (Charge 2).

Recommendation 1. The Department of Defense (DoD), the branches of the armed services, and the Department of Veterans Affairs (DVA) should continue to work together to develop, fund, and staff medical information systems that include a single, uniform, continuous, and retrievable electronic medical record for each service person. The uniform record should include each relevant health item (including baseline personal risk factors, every inpatient and outpatient medical contact, and all health-related interventions), allow linkage to exposure and other data sets, and have the capability to incorporate relevant medical data from beyond DoD and DVA institutions (e.g., U.S. Public Health Service facilities, civilian medical providers, and other health care institutions). Appropriate consent and protection of individual privacy must be considered for information obtained and included.

Finding

The number and variety of studies regarding consequences of the PGW are already considerable. To date, most health-related studies specifically involving PGW veterans have focused on short-term mental health consequences of deployment, the role of combat exposure, and other stressors experienced in the theater of operations and, to a lesser extent, on problems relating to demobilization and readjustment to civilian life among reservist and National Guard personnel. A few reports have included limited longitudinal follow-up data concerning men and women who served in the PG. Important information may be gained through longer follow-up of some of these groups, particularly since at least one of these groups was first to arrive in the theater, and precombat data are available. Also needed are studies of risk factors in modern deployments predictive of combat stress reactions, posttraumatic stress disorder (PTSD), and other psychiatric disorders of military personnel and veterans. Studies relevant to the trauma of war and the ensuing mental health consequences should concentrate special attention on improving efforts in prevention, intervention, and follow-up (Charge 3).

Recommendation 2. The DoD and DVA should conduct further studies, with appropriate statistical and epidemiological support, to identify risk factors for stress-related psychiatric disorders among military personnel (active and reserve) and to develop better methods to buffer and ameliorate the psychiatric consequences of modern training, deployment, combat, demobilization, and return to daily living.

Recommendation 3. Studies being conducted by DoD and DVA that have included longitudinal follow-up of the mental health of veterans who served in the PG should be supported with continued follow-up after appropriate peer review of study methods. Follow-up in these studies should be sufficient to provide at least a decade of information comparing the mental health status of those deployed with those not deployed.

Finding

The military dominance of U.S. forces in the PGW increased the relative significance of physical and natural environmental exposures as important sources of potential morbidity and mortality, compared with combat injuries. This is likely to recur in future deployments (Charge 2).

Recommendation 4. The DoD should ensure that military medical preparedness for deployments includes detailed attempts to monitor natural and man-made environmental exposures and to prepare for rapid response, early investigation, and accurate data collection, when possible, on physical and natural environmental exposures that are known or possible in the specific theater of operations.

Finding

National Guard and reserve component personnel may differ substantially from active duty personnel in average age, level of training, occupational specialties, family status, and readiness for deployment. Further, it is unclear whether either policies and procedures or the manner in which they are implemented differs between activated reserve or National Guard units and active duty troops for mobilization, deployment, demobilization, and return. All of these factors may affect the health consequences of deployment (Charge 3).

Recommendation 5. Research is needed to determine whether differences in personal characteristics or differences in policies and procedures for mobilization, deployment, demobilization, and return of reserves, National Guard, and regular troops are associated with different or adverse health consequences. If there are associations, strategies necessary to prevent or reduce these adverse health effects should be developed.

Finding

Completed studies have described the mortality experience of troops deployed to the PG during the period of deployment and in the 2-year period after deployment. These studies have documented a consistent pattern of increased risk of death from unintentional injury for the cohort of deployed troops compared with those not deployed to the PG. However, death rates from disease were not significantly increased. Continued monitoring and further study of mortality rates among veterans of the PGW will be of value in assessing the long-term health consequences of deployment (Charge 3).

Recommendation 6. The mortality experience of PG veterans should continue to be monitored for as long as 30 years, on a regular basis, including comparisons with that of PG-era veterans. (PG-era veterans have been defined as those in military service at the time of the PGW, but assigned or deployed elsewhere.) Research investigators should focus on the reported excess mortality from unintentional injury, on mortality from specific illnesses, and on evidence of elevation (or reduction) in the risk of death from other causes.

Recommendation 7. The DVA should exert greater effort to improve understanding of the reasons for excess mortality from unintentional injury. Detailed evaluation is needed beyond death certificate data concerning the circumstances surrounding fatal injury through more focused case-control studies to identify both individual risk factors and remediable causes.

Finding

The armed services and the DVA together are developing a shared basic epidemiological data system, the Defense Medical Epidemiological Database (DMED) (Charge 2).

Recommendation 8. The DMED system should be continued, expanded as planned, expedited to develop the proposed integrated information management system, linked to other key systems, and evaluated regularly.

Finding

Considerable effort has been devoted by DoD to the development of a Troop Exposure Assessment Model (TEAM) for describing the PGW experience of veterans. This has included the completion of an information system designed to establish the geographic location of each unit from January 15, 1991, until the unit departed from the Gulf theater. This system has the potential to be linked to data on regional environmental conditions but will necessarily be devoid of most individual data (such as pesticide exposure or individual health risk factors) (Charge 2).

Recommendation 9. The DoD should complete development of information systems to expeditiously and directly pinpoint unit locations at a high level of disaggregation in space and time (that is, fine detail) and to document local environmental conditions, including appropriate data quality checks, with direct data entry into the system. There is likely to be a need for a similar information system during and after any future conflict, and DoD should prepare and continually update plans for such a nonpaper system. A manual for use of the information systems by research investigators should be compiled, with the strengths and limitations identified.

Finding

The power and complexity of analyses based on space-time geographical information system (GIS) data require careful attention to data quality and the limits imposed by various data items. Quality improvement and assessment of limits are continuous processes and depend on detailed evaluation of data needs for specific analytic questions (Charge 2).

Recommendation 10. For every specific question posed to the current TEAM, DoD should assess the strengths and limitations of the TEAM as a resource for evaluating the health significance of geographically defined exposures of troops, including those in the PGW and those in conflicts that may develop in the future. Evaluations and recommendations for possible modification of the TEAM should be reported to the PG Coordinating Board, Research Working Group.

Finding

Given the unprecedented numbers of women serving in the PG, especially those in largely new roles, including combat support, it is important to specially evaluate the health consequences and needs for health services of women who served in the PG. Preliminary findings from studies being conducted at the Boston VA Medical Center (VAMC) indicate that additional research in this area is needed. Additional research is also needed on the health effects of having male and female personnel serve together in combat or under threat of combat (Charge 3).

Recommendation 11. The DoD and DVA should ensure that studies of the health effects of deployment, including effects on PGW veterans, include evaluation of exposures, experiences, and situations of both women and men, with attention to their age, prior military service, marital and parental status, and other gender-specific parameters.

Recommendation 12. The DoD and DVA should conduct studies of the health consequences of assigning men and women to serve together in combat or under the threat of enemy action. Such work should be undertaken with a focus on prevention and amelioration of any added stresses.

Finding

Several important studies are currently under way. Worthwhile data are being collected and prepared, and the studies should be completed promptly, with the necessary personnel and funding to collect the additional data needed, to conduct appropriate analyses, and to evaluate potential biases. Findings from these studies are likely to provide leads as to whether or not additional research along these lines is required to produce more specific findings (Charges 1 and 3).

• The Naval Health Research Center at San Diego has undertaken a series of studies under the general title of "Epidemiologic Studies of Morbidity Among Gulf War Veterans: A Search for Etiologic Agents and Risk Factors." These studies hold promise for answering some important questions about the health of PGW veterans after demobilization and about the possibility that veterans and their spouses may experience an excess risk of adverse pregnancy outcomes as a result of service in the PGW. The studies are being carried out with care, excellent planning, and proper pilot efforts to determine feasibility. Upon completion, these studies should provide important guidance concerning whether veterans have experienced hospitalization at rates in excess of their nondeployed peers, have developed specific symptoms or illnesses related to their PGW experience, or have experienced risks that have resulted in adverse reproductive outcomes related to their service in the Gulf.

Recommendation 13a. The Naval Health Research studies in San Diego should be completed and results published as designed and scheduled.

• Although there are significant problems with the DVA National Health Survey, the investigators have designed additional phases of the study that will be important to complete. The physical examinations and follow-up of nonrespondents to the mail survey will be an important step toward describing potential biases and evaluating signs and symptoms of both PG and PG-era study participants.

Recommendation 13b. The DVA National Health Survey should be completed and results published as designed and scheduled.

• The DVA-DoD study that was designed to examine predictors of enrollment in the DVA PG Health Registry (PGHR) may provide useful information as to what objectively measurable factors contribute to self-selection into the registry. In addition to the proposed analysis of associations among demographics, past health experiences, and health behaviors as possible predictors of enrollment, information on the eligibility of individuals for health care, as well as the type of health care, could generate additional hypotheses to be investigated.

Recommendation 13c. Evaluation of predictors of enrollment in the DVA PGHR should be promptly completed and results published. Included, if possible. should be information on type of care requested, required, and received.

Finding

The armed forces have had small but high-quality and effective capabilities in epidemiology. Recent cutbacks have reduced these capabilities, with potentially serious effects on both military preparedness and the health care of veterans. The Theater Area Medical Laboratory (TAML) is an example of how specialists can respond rapidly to potential health problems of troops deployed in various areas of the world and provide immediate and useful information necessary to maintain the military readiness of the armed forces. In addition, well-trained epidemiologists and preventive medicine specialists are necessary for conducting the relevant population-based epidemiologic studies, with comprehensive exposure assessment, that have the greatest likelihood of being informative about the health consequences of any future deployment. Such capability should permit studies that extend beyond the time of an individual's active duty service and that are capable of responding to questions of delayed effects that may emerge only years, or even decades, after a military operation (Charge 1).

Recommendation 14. The epidemiologic capabilities of the armed forces should be strengthened rather than reduced. The command structure should be kept informed about the reasons for and the results of this recommendation and its relevance to military preparedness and effectiveness, and should be encouraged to support appropriate epidemiologic work in the theater of operations and in the postdeployment period.

Finding

Much good work on symptom complexes and other matters discussed in this report has been done by DoD, DVA, and their contractors. However, it is evident from the references cited in this report that many are in the "gray literature"—available to those who know they exist and how to ask for them, but not published in the open, peer-reviewed scientific literature where they will be fully indexed and readily available, with some assurance that they meet at least minimal scientific standards. Even this committee, with the contacts and expertise it developed over time, had difficulty in identifying and obtaining some of these reports. The committee also is concerned about the high cost of much recent research and the necessity for maximizing the nation's overall return on that investment. In summary, the committee believes that health-related research is not finalized until it is published and readily accessible in peer-reviewed journals (Charge 1).

Recommendation 15. The DoD and DVA should adopt a policy that internal and contract-supported reports on health research will be submitted for publication in the peer-reviewed scientific literature in a timely manner.

Finding

Some research directed toward reports of unexplained illnesses after the PGW was flawed in the questions posed, populations studied, or research design. We believe that these defects could have been identified before research projects were funded if requests for proposals had been announced generally and had been open to the scientific community at large and if fully developed research proposals had been reviewed by panels of qualified expert peers. Some research was announced and reviewed in this manner, but much more could be so treated, to the benefit of both veterans and the public (Charge 1).

Recommendation 16. The Congress, DVA, and DoD should adopt a policy that unless there are well-specified, openly stated reasons to the contrary, requests for proposals for research related to unexplained illnesses or other needed health-related research will be publicly announced and open to the scientific community at large, that proposals will be reviewed by panels of appropriately qualified experts, and that funding will follow the recommendations of those experts.

3

Environment and Exposures

OVERVIEW

There have been special concerns about a range of both naturally occurring and either purposeful or accidental environmental exposures of troops during the Persian Gulf War (PGW) that are discussed in this chapter.

Objective indicators of harmful environmental exposures in the Persian Gulf (PG) were limited in scope during the PGW and are not readily usable for research purposes. Monitors of air and soil contaminants were not operating for the full period of Operation Desert Shield/Storm (ODS/S), and other kinds of exposures were not measured. Exposure indicators of other than air or soil were not available. Autopsies of animals and humans and follow-up examinations of military working dogs (MWDs) have not indicated the presence of excessive toxic or heavy metals, particularly when data before and after the oil well fires are compared. Official reports of acute health consequences from exposure to air pollutants were rare.

It is clear from written descriptions and reports by veterans that the PG was a hostile environment. Desert conditions, the absence of amenities, uncomfortable temperatures and humidities, extremes in rainfall, blowing sand, insects, animals, fumes, and smoke—all contributed to adverse living conditions. In addition, wartime conditions, including measures uniquely designed to protect the troops, necessitated other exposures such as vaccines against possible biological warfare (BW) agents, pyridostigmine bromide (PB) to protect against possible chemical warfare (CW) agents, and pesticides to protect against bites from insects carrying diseases such as sandfly fever and leishmaniasis. Depleted uranium (DU), used in munitions and tank armor, was a limited but real wartime exposure. Unfortunately, there was no systematic accumulation of data on these exposures, making research into their possible health effects exceptionally difficult, if not impossible.

In the midst of these adverse environmental and wartime-related exposures, soldiers were vulnerable to all of the exposures connected with their particular occupations in the Gulf, such as chemical-agent-resistant coatings (CARCs), solvents, and vehicle exhaust fumes. Information about "unofficial" exposures, such as the combustion products of leaded fuels in heaters that were sometimes unventilated or nonregulation, wearing flea collars to protect against insect bites, and ingesting alcohol substitutes in the absence of approved alcohol consumption is available only from self-reports.

Not surprisingly, the above scenario creates a picture of an extremely stressful environment, filled with the dangers and trauma of war, combined with a hostile living and work environment. Contributing to this stress were the lack of sanitary conditions and privacy (particularly when men and women were serving together); the speed of being "called-up" to duty and thrown into this environment; "watchful waiting" for the shooting war to begin or SCUD missiles to explode; apprehension heightened by drills and training exercises relating to the threat of chemical and biological warfare (CBW); intense workloads; and sleep deprivation. Additionally, issues related to unit cohesion, leadership, morale, and knowledge of family stresses back home varied among individuals but are important for full understanding of the experience of the entire deployed cohort.

Although a wide range of possible exposures might be associated with adverse health outcomes in PG veterans, data on these exposures are often not available; when they are available, they are poorly documented. This lack of exposure information is at the core of the frustration in obtaining answers from epidemiologic studies. Self-reports of exposure and estimates of individual exposure from unit-level measurements will be subject to so much error that they are likely to yield inconclusive results and additional questions.

This situation leads us to recommend improvements in collecting data on exposure assessment in future military deployments. We divide our more detailed discussion of exposures into two broad categories: the physical environment, which includes both the natural and the man-made environments, and psychosocial exposures. Generally, it is relatively straightforward to list potential causative agents, but exposure estimates related to PGW operations are crude and unreliable. Efforts are under way to obtain additional estimates and improve current estimates, but there is little potential for substantial improvement.

The working conditions and exposures that veterans encountered in the PG include the natural environment of the PGW theater of operations, as well as occupational and combat-related exposures and situational stresses that combine all of the aforementioned. The environment and exposures of interest included those enumerated earlier, as well as dirt, sanitary conditions, endemic infectious diseases, flora and fauna, oil well spills and fires, pesticides, oil and petroleum products (especially jet fuel and diesel fuel containing lead additives), mycotoxins, and decontamination solutions. Occupational exposures were related mainly to general maintenance operations and include battery repair, cleaning and degreasing, electronic and radio repair, generator repair, grinding and sanding, sandblasting, lathing and milling, painting (especially with isocyanate-based paints), refrigeration servicing, vehicle repair, weapons repair, and welding and cutting. Work shifts were often longer than peacetime work schedules (e.g., 12–16 hours), with fewer "time-off" periods (e.g., weekends and holidays), so that permissible exposure levels based on 8-hour shifts may not afford protection similar to that in civilian settings.

The environment also was made more complex by the exposure of a large number of troops to potentially life-saving vaccinations, to medications administered in an effort to protect troops from chemical warfare (e.g., pyridostigmine), to clothing treated with permethrin, and to insect repellents (especially *N*, *N*-diethyl-*m*-toluamide [Deet]). All of this took place in a background of the barrage of news reports that reinforced the unknown nature of the threat the soldiers faced. The possibility of CBW was considered very real; most combatants expected the Iraqis to launch attacks by missiles containing both explosives and chemical or biological weapons. In addition, some accustomed ways of relieving stress were simply absent. For example, interchange with the indigenous population was almost entirely forbidden, and there were severe restrictions on the availability of alcoholic beverages. The ease of communication with home, while in certain respects providing emotional support, also served to keep some people focused on what they had left, as well as on their current task. Finally, the level of casualties was very low; the lack of battle casualties in the PG may have diminished the possibility of rationalizing an acceptable trauma as a way to explain puzzling tensions and anxieties. The absence of this traditional military avenue for both experience and release of stress, and for explanation of the psychological symptoms being experienced, may have unmasked emotional conflicts that were perhaps harder to understand than when or if they had been experienced in previous conflicts.

Thus, service personnel stationed in the Gulf were exposed to an extraordinary array of environmental conditions. Their complex experiences combined to yield what is truly a varied and sometimes confusing picture of exposure that has proven difficult to understand, much less reconstruct. Herein, we delineate the relevant exposures by reviewing available data, recognizing that these exposures combined to produce an environment that is more complex than can be easily described or evaluated.

NATURAL ENVIRONMENT

Characteristics of the natural environment in the PG were discussed in the committee's first report and are summarized as follows. Mean daily low and high temperatures, respectively, were 80°F and 108°F in July (temperatures could reach 130°F on a summer day [Young et al., 1992]) and 45°F and 65°F in the winter in the coastal region. Temperatures in the northwest desert were reported to be lower. Except in coastal regions, the relative humidity was less than 40% during the summer (less than 6% inland [Young et al., 1992]), but more than 60% during the rainy season (December through March). Solar heat was intense in the summer. Rain was minimal but sometimes caused tents to flood.

Many troops were located in desert settings. Sand was ubiquitous and often powdery, and persons with respiratory conditions sometimes reported pulmonary symptoms. Whether these symptoms were properly attributed to sand rather than to the type of living structure (tent versus air-conditioned building) or other problems has not been determined (Richards et al., 1993b).

Review of sanitation in the PG theater is not currently possible from available records. The following has been reported as a summary of the sanitary conditions (O'Donnell, 1994):

> Staging areas near ports of entry were characterized by crowded tent living with strains on latrine facilities, showers, and feeding. The prototype four-seat latrines were mass produced by contract in country. Latrines were designed for suction removal of waste by contractors or burn-out. Early designs permitted ingress of flies. In the desert environment, daily burning out of waste cans employed mainly diesel fuel. Smoke from such fires was common, though rapidly dispersed by prevailing winds. Solid waste disposal was handled by contract in the staging areas and by burning in pits in the desert. Locations for burn pits and latrines were usually chosen carefully to minimize nuisance from smoke, smells, and flies. When shower/bath units were not available, many field expedients were improvised. Likewise for laundry. As shower setups became available or were improvised, an unforeseen problem was heating the water once the cooler weather set in. Time intervals between showers and uniform laundering were sometimes lengthy.

Anecdotal reports suggest that living and working areas were subject to smoke from waste fires for the duration of the fire. Efforts to minimize the nuisance of latrines and burn pits were not always successful because of wind shifts.

The possibility that troops were exposed to contaminated water or food was low, because local drinking water was processed and treated before use. Troops were usually provided with sealed containers of drinking water; food was provided at mess halls or as a meal ready-to-eat (MRE) sealed in plastic; personnel generally did not eat food produced in local areas.

An exposure of concern to troops in the PGW was the bite of the sand fly, which may carry the parasite that causes leishmaniasis and sandfly fever. Many cases of cutaneous leishmaniasis were expected, and a small number were in fact observed. What had not been expected was the appearance of a new manifestation of leishmaniasis caused by *Leishmania tropica* (Magill et al., 1993; MMWR, 1992); *L. tropica* usually causes cutaneous disease but was described with visceral symptoms as viscerotropic leishmaniasis. Visceral leishmaniasis usually is caused by *L. donovani,* but exposures during ODS/S included *L. tropica,* which is hard to detect and makes the diagnosis or exclusion of leishmaniasis more difficult. At least 12 cases of visceral disease have been reported, but diagnosis is difficult and requires isolation of the parasite from bone marrow and no sufficiently selective and specific serology and skin tests have yet been developed. It has been postulated by some that this new form of the disease may be an explanation for some of the undiagnosed illnesses in PGW veterans.

The committee's first report recommended support of continued research on leishmaniasis, especially to develop improved techniques for diagnosis, and further study of the ecology of the disease. Both the Department of Veterans Affairs (DVA) and the Department of Defense (DoD) have continued to support basic scientific research in response to these recommendations (see Appendix F), particularly the development of a skin test to diagnose leishmaniasis.

Other exposures to fauna also have been described (O'Donnell, 1994):

> Filth flies were a universal problem in the warm months. Latrines and food sources were attractants. The use of screening, self-closing doors, fly traps, fly bait, and pesticides were moderately successful suppressants. Various types of scorpions and snakes such as the horned viper were common in the desert, and envenomation of personnel occurred occasionally. Although biting spiders were present, they were not a problem. Mosquitoes were a factor only in the Euphrates Valley. Sand flies were present, as evidenced by the cases of leishmaniasis, but were difficult to find even when searched for. Sheep and camels were commonly observed in the desert. Dead sheep were often reported, but veterinary inquiries disclosed no signs of unexpected causes of death. Unit pets or mascots were officially banned but some small units adopted stray dogs and obtained veterinary care through Saudi sources.

There have been numerous and persistent reports in presentations by individuals who were present during the PGW of finding large numbers of dead sheep, goats, camels, and other animals in the region. One published report assessed the histopathologic and chemical analysis of 26 feral cats exposed to the Kuwait oil fires (Moeller et al., 1994); the analysis concluded that there was little evidence of harm from the environment. This has engendered some concern that the cause of death of these animals was chemical and/or biological weapons used in the Gulf at the time of the war. Additionally, veterinarians in Kuwait found no animal deaths due to chemical or biological weapon use, although many animals were killed by Iraqi soldiers and many died from water deprivation. In an effort to evaluate this matter further, the committee has attempted to locate and review as much relevant material as possible, including internal documents of the U.S. armed services that were generated both at the time of the PGW and later.

The Army was well aware at the outset of the PGW that zoonotic diseases could be a major issue. Defense against chemical and biological weapons was a high priority. As a result, Army veterinarians, Air Force Special Operations Medical Officers, Army Chemical Warfare Specialists, and physicians specializing in infectious diseases were in the theater to evaluate any unusual animal deaths. An investigation of thousands of dead sheep was conducted early in Operation Desert Storm (ODS) after dead animals had been observed in various locations and at different times by Army medical personnel. The team estimated that the animals had been dead for various periods, ranging from days to months. Several investigative teams concluded that the areas in which the animals were found seemed to be dumping grounds for those that had succumbed to indigenous bacterial illness. Biological samples from this site were analyzed by the U.S. Army Medical Research Institute of Infectious Diseases (USAMRIID) and found to be negative for anthrax. Other reports of dead sheep were received but were not investigated due to poor weather conditions and inadequate description of the location of the dead animals. However, the U.S. agriculture attaché advised military authorities that a 5–10 percent death rate from endemic infectious agents in sheep was common and that dead sheep were routinely stacked along common roadways to allow government inspectors to check ear tags and arrange for indemnity payments. This information was disseminated to U.S. Army veterinarians, and based on a lack of clinical signs in animals grazing nearby, no further clinical investigations were conducted during ODS. During the ground war, one on-site investigation of dead sheep was conducted and was negative for chemical or biological weapon use.

After the war, discussions with local veterinarians confirmed that the practice of placing dead sheep by roadsides is common. Local practitioners have been consistently unaware of any unusual occurrences of death of sheep during or after ODS. Veterinarians and other medical personnel reported nearly unanimously that animal deaths from enzootic disease and trauma were common on the open range, even in the absence of military forces. These enzootic diseases are not known to be transmitted to people under the circumstances that existed during ODS/S (Stevens, 1995).

Approximately 140 MWDs were deployed to various locations in the PG (Dutton, 1995). Since the PGW, 31 of these dogs have been euthanized because of arthritis, senility, cancer, temperament, multiple organ failure, and visual or inner ear problems; 5 died of natural causes (1 of heart failure and 4 of twisted stomach). No evidence of unusual morbidity or mortality was reported.

The committee reviewed a protocol for a study of 129 MWDs identified as deployed to the Gulf between August 1, 1990, and February 28, 1991. From this cohort of deployed dogs, pathological specimens will be examined for approximately 20 MWDs that had died or been humanely euthanized and approximately 20 matched MWDs that had not been deployed to the Gulf. Additionally, MWDs deployed to the Gulf will be compared to a similar number not deployed to the Gulf (including follow-up until death or humane euthanasia) for pathologic, clinical, and demographic differences.

MAN-MADE ENVIRONMENT

Pesticides

Reports to this and other panels (such as the DVA's PG Expert Scientific Panel) have been made on the use and safety of pesticides in the PG and in general (Berté, 1994). The pesticides available in the PG during ODS/S included (in pounds) malathion (45,770), chlorpyrifos (8,410), D-phenothrin (1,858), methomyl (903), and lindane (539). Pyrethrin, dichlorvos (DDVP), carbaryl, propoxur, and diazinon were also available but in amounts less than 330 pounds. It is not known how much of this inventory of pesticides was actually used or what troop exposures may have resulted (Bolton, 1995).

The use of pesticides in the Gulf was reported to have followed strict guidelines (Bolton, 1995). They were used only after arthropod surveys that identified individual pests and estimated arthropod prevalence. Distribution of pesticides was prohibited unless approved by the local commander. Distribution or use for other than personal purposes was restricted to trained or certified personnel or contractors. There were some reports by troops of rash from misuse of dog flea collars.

The insect repellent permethrin was used to treat uniforms in the PG; the material used to make the uniforms used during ODS/S was not pretreated in the factory with permethrin. Some troops were reported to have both used Deet on their skin and treated their clothing with permethrin between August and October 1990 (the peak occurrence of arthropods). From October 1990 to February 1991, the need for Deet and permethrin decreased as the population of arthropods declined (Bolton, 1995).

Personal application of the insect repellent (33 percent Deet) provided to soldiers for use on the skin has been calculated based on the amount of repellent ordered for the Gulf operation and the amount returned (Bolton, 1995). An average of approximately 2.7 tubes of repellent was available for use per soldier. The recommended deployment issue was two tubes per person, with each 60-ml tube containing an estimated 24 applications, or enough for approximately 12 days. Similar calculations indicate an average of 0.1 bottle (2 ounces) of 75 percent Deet per soldier to be used for personal application to clothing; this material could also have been applied to skin.

The virtual absence of reports of sandfly fever (Richards et al., 1991) and negative findings for sandfly fever in tests of pre- and postdeployment sera (Richards et al., 1993a) suggest that vector control was generally good. This inference has been reinforced in reports that the deployed troops had no known outbreaks of sandfly fever, no evidence of typhus or spotted fever-group rickettsia infection, 1 case of West Nile fever, 20 cases of cutaneous leishmaniasis, 12 cases of visceral leishmaniasis, and 7 cases of malaria (Bolton, 1995; Hyams et al., 1995).

There has been some concern about the delayed effects of pesticide exposure. This concern is particularly prominent for organophosphorus pesticides, which have been reported to be associated with a delayed neurotoxicity (Abou-Donia and Lapadula, 1990). The early biochemical events associated with organophosphate-induced delayed neurotoxicity (OPIDN) remain unidentified. There are striking species differences in susceptibility to OPIDN, as well as differences in the potency of organophosphate compounds (Abou-Donia and Lapadula, 1990). Where comparative assays have been developed, the chicken is a commonly used model system to assess the potency of compounds to induce OPIDN (Abou-Donia and Lapadula, 1990). In humans, symptoms of neurologic dysfunction typically begin within 2 weeks of cessation of overexposure. Patients generally complain initially of symmetric lower extremity weakness, with subsequent progression lasting 3–6 months after onset of symptoms. The patient may then enter a "stationary" phase of the illness, often lasting 3–12 months. Improvement may be observed 6–18 months after onset of initial symptoms. Even in the most severe cases, there is usually improvement in the upper extremity impairment. Spinal cord damage can be permanent in the most severely affected patients.

Specific agents have been studied to determine their ability to induce this condition. Chlorpyrifos, one of the pesticides used in the PGW, was reviewed recently by Richardson (1995), who concluded that exposure as a result of "normal use" is unlikely to result in OPIDN. However, a report of eight cases of reversible neurologic disease in individuals with an exposure to an unknown amount of chlorpyrifos has raised some concern that a mild reversible sensory neuropathology may be associated with subchronic administration. In general, it appears that the average personal usage of the pesticides available in the PGW theater of operations was low and unlikely to be associated with the induction of chronic disease.

Fuels and Decontamination Solution

Many different fuels were used in the PG both for vehicles and for heaters, cooking stoves, and portable generators. The exhaust produced by these fuels (particularly the reported use of unventilated heaters in living quarters that might have contained mixtures of diesel and jet fuel) could have caused a variety of exposures to combustion products, including lead. Information received in response to a request to DoD on whether leaded fuel was used in tent heaters stated that U.S. Central Command records indicated that approximately 145,000 gallons of gasoline (leaded and from local sources) were consumed per day in the theater between August 1, 1990, and March 30, 1991. These records did not indicate whether the fuel was used for heating tents; it was intended for use in vehicles, cooking, and power generation. The individual services provided information on the use of leaded gasoline in tent heaters as follows: Air Force, electric heat exclusively; Navy, kerosene and diesel fuel only; Marine Corps, diesel only; Army, "has no record of leaded fuel use in tent heaters" (Cusick, 1996).

To investigate further possible effects from this exposure, in combination with other exposures that were prevalent at various times in the Gulf, DoD has funded a laboratory study in rats to evaluate the toxicity of simulated PGW exposures. This research initiative has as its chief aim the investigation of rodent responses to exposure conditions similar to those experienced by PGW veterans. In an effort to construct a rodent model of unexplained illness in PGW veterans, Sprague-Dawley rats will be subjected to controlled experimental exposure to Deet, pyridostigmine, and a mixture of diesel and jet fuel followed by an electrical shock; controls will help to delineate possible effects of chamber exposures alone, compared with exposures with stress-producing electrical shock. Postexposure testing will include examination of central nervous system (CNS) integrity (auditory startle and adaptation to auditory stimulus and photosensitivity), testing of motor skills (grip and total activity), neurotransmitter analysis at sacrifice, two-dimensional gel electrophoresis to investigate whether novel stress-related proteins are produced in stressed animals, clinical chemistry, and measures of immune function.

This ambitious protocol, as reviewed, may produce hypothesis-generating data. However, generalization of any results to veterans will necessarily be problematic. No variation in dosing will be done, and no dose-rate considerations are included. Although these animals are useful models for some known human conditions, the applicability of any adverse (or the opposite) outcomes noted in these studies will inevitably be questioned.

Oil Well Fires and Spills

Many agencies were involved in monitoring and measuring various aspects of the oil well fires and smoke (EPA, 1991; U.S. Gulf Environmental Technical Assistance, 1992; WMO, 1991, 1992). Several efforts have been made to determine whether the oil well fires and spills created by retreating Iraqi forces affected the health of U.S. troops (DoD, 1993; USAEHA, 1992, 1994). One major effort at environmental assessment and health impact was undertaken by the former U.S. Army Environmental Hygiene Agency (USAEHA), currently known as the U.S. Army Center for Health Promotion and Preventive Medicine (USACHPPM). Although exposures began when the first oil well fires were ignited by the Iraqi armed forces during their retreat in February 1991, and some lasted until November 1, 1991, USAEHA could not launch a successful air-sampling effort until the beginning of May, after the more stagnant air conditions of the winter months had passed. Those who undertook the sampling efforts did so with this knowledge. They intended to address the problem as thoroughly as possible by the use of meteorological modeling. A geographical information system (GIS) is being developed to integrate information over space and time on airborne and soil-based exposures, on meteorological conditions throughout the study interval, and on unit troop movements during ODS. Once this model is available, exposure of individual troops can be estimated throughout the region, although further work will still be needed to validate the model and estimate its precision.

There were as many as 10 fixed air-sampling stations in the theater, but 2 of them operated for less than 2 weeks and 2 more operated for only 2 months. Three were in operation through the end of December 1991. These fixed sites were located where troops were concentrated, and soil was sampled from the same areas. The results are to be combined with National Oceanic and Atmospheric Administration (NOAA)-assisted modeling and records of troop movements using the GIS to estimate reasonable maximum individual exposures (RMEs) to the chemical substances sampled. Data available include air and soil pathway analysis and industrial hygiene sampling. Air and soil quality was estimated not to have deteriorated during the sampling interval, and a reference to earlier sampling suggests that air quality at some sites was even higher than before the war. Increases in toxic metals in soil were not found during sampling except for metals unrelated to Kuwaiti crude oil.

Air pollutants expected from the oil fires were classified into four categories: reactants (uncombusted crude oil components), combustion products (e.g., carbon dioxide and water), incomplete combustion products (e.g., carbon monoxide), and products of secondary reactions (photolysis). The substances included short-chain and low to medium molecular weight aliphatics such as butane and heptane (both straight and branched chain) in the range of C_2 to C_{40}, simple and polycyclic aromatic hydrocarbons (PAHs), benzene, heterocyclic compounds including naphthalene and xylene, and substituted compounds such as methylated and halogenated compounds. Air samples were assayed for suspended particulates, both total and less than 10 μm in diameter, and for a series of volatile organics, PAHs, and metals. A subsample was examined for sulfur dioxide, nitrogen dioxide, coal-tar pitch volatiles, and acid aerosols. These agents were chosen as likely to provide a reasonable estimate of the most important particulates of the oil well fires and spills. The sampling was designed so that results could be used to estimate risks of cancer and subchronic noncancer diseases.

So far, based on our present knowledge, none of the individual agents sampled or detected seems likely to cause symptoms that would persist for months or years after return from the PG. However, the modeling now in progress may offer some improved understanding of the general environment of troops located in different parts of the war zone or may raise questions about interactive effects or combined exposures.

The USAEHA sampling (after May 1991) documented little deterioration of general air quality during that period of air monitoring. Although substantial increases were noted in particulates, concentrations were still considered "normal" for this area of the Middle East. Exposures to organic compounds were similar to levels observed in Houston and Philadelphia, cities with major petrochemical industries. There were relatively high concentrations of naturally occurring metals, apparently from wind-blown surface soils.

There was some concern about ingestion and dermal absorption of air pollutants that had settled out, and these routes of exposure have been considered (USAEHA, 1994). However, no measurements were taken, so possible exposures through these additional routes can be estimated only by mathematical models.

Further work by USAEHA is expected to provide a model of exposure distributions and to incorporate information from earlier, more limited sampling that might improve estimates of exposures at troop encampments. This work also will examine the frequency and duration of exposures. The model will have to be validated and its precision estimated before evaluating the relevance of the data.

The Armed Forces Institute of Pathology (AFIP) has completed a study of 351 autopsies of U.S. personnel who died between August 1990 and November 1991 in Southwest Asia (SWA) during ODS/S and shortly thereafter. Reviewed were written autopsy records, histopathologic specimens, and toxicologic findings. A group of 149 individuals who died before the oil fires were lit was compared with a group of 202 who died after the fires were lit. No evidence was found to support an association between autopsy, histopathologic, and toxicologic findings and any environmental exposures, including smoke from oil well fires. Analysis for heavy metals from blood and tissue obtained at autopsy did not indicate elevated levels attributable to exposure in the Gulf environment (Peterson and Kalasinsky, 1996). The initial findings (AFIP, 1994) reviewed by this committee indicated that lead levels were elevated in some of the specimens (IOM, 1995a). Since that time, investigators from AFIP have stated that with respect to lead, no valid toxicological conclusions can be drawn because some specimens were reportedly drawn and stored in collection vessels containing lead. The methods and findings of this study are being prepared for submission to a peer-reviewed journal.

Occupational Exposures

Little information has been identified characterizing the range of occupational exposures that may have occurred in the PG beyond those associated with the occupation of "soldier." It appears that the majority of occupational chemical exposures were related to repair and maintenance activities. No information is currently available on the numbers of troops who were assigned regularly or intermittently to the different components of support work in the PG.

Table 3-1 includes most of the potential chemical hazards associated with common maintenance or repair operations. With the exception of vehicle painting, information on actual exposure evaluations for these work settings is not available.

Table 3-1. Potential Chemical Hazards Associated with Common Maintenance or Repair Operations

Operation	Chemical Hazard(s)
Battery repair	Corrosive liquids, particularly sulfuric acid; lead
Cleaning/degreasing	Solvents generally, including a range of chlorinated hydrocarbons such as trichloroethylene
Electronic/radio repair	Soldering fumes and cleaning solvents
Generator repair	Carbon monoxide
Grinding/sanding	Abrasive particulates
Lathing/milling	Metalworking fluids
Refrigeration servicing	Lead fumes and exposure to refrigerants such as fluorocarbons
Sandblasting	Abrasive particulates (possibly including crystalline silica) in the respirable range
Vehicle painting	Paint solvent vapors and mists
Vehicle repair	Asbestos from brake repair, carbon monoxide, organic solvents
Weapons repair	Lead particulates
Welding/cutting	Chromates, ozone, nitrogen dioxide, and heated metal fumes

Because operating conditions were far from ideal and the environments generally were not sufficiently fixed for adherence to recommended occupational hygiene controls, some of these exposures could have been substantial. Trained industrial hygienists stationed in the Gulf reported that exposures in fixed work environments generally could have been kept within current standards, but that operations in the field may not have allowed sufficiently stringent controls (Riley, 1992). This was particularly the case for painting operations that called for exposure control in painting operations. The industrial hygiene staff used the American Conference of Governmental Industrial Hygienists' (ACGIH) Threshold Limit Values (TLVs) as their primary guide. Commentary indicates that these limits were considered sufficient to protect against health effects (USAEHA, 1992). However, many of these limits are based on feasibility rather than on protecting against all health effects (Rappaport, 1993).

Initial and repair painting operations created a potential for overexposure to isocyanate paints, which can cause primary sensitization and asthma as well as exacerbation of existing asthma. The CARC paint system was used directly by an estimated 1,000 troops (PGVCB, 1994). The number of vehicles painted each day varied between 10 and 100 at the major work site in Al Jabayl. At least one episode of overexposure (December 1990) was reported (Riley, 1992).

USAEHA industrial hygiene sampling showed increases in personal or general air monitoring results of outdoor occupational environment from selected times and locations, but these increased levels did not exceed recommended standards. The relevance of these times and locations to the exposures of troops is not known.

Overall, although the committee has been unable to find evidence that occupational exposures caused serious or frequent health problems, the possibility cannot be ruled out.

Diet

During the PGW, troops were issued prepackaged meals known as MREs. There were 12 varieties of MREs, each meal consisting of six to eight foods that were approved for 10 days of continuous use. Another committee of the Institute of Medicine (IOM) has recently released a report that discusses the issues of using MREs for longer than recommended periods; inadequate nutrition resulting from less that the required number of calories and nutrients; types of foods that receive higher acceptance; inclusion of supplemental packs to improve acceptability; and evaluation of the MRE for use under adverse conditions (IOM, 1995c). The report found that underconsumption of approximately 1,552 kcal/day relative to measured energy expenditure was demonstrated. One of the research areas suggested by that report related to how MRE food item wastage affects specific nutrient intake and the relation between energy intake and expenditure. The report indicates that changes have been made since the PGW in the composition of MREs to improve the quality of the meals, as well as the likelihood of consumption. The military now uses an MRE that is certified for use for 30 days. A recently formed IOM committee is undertaking a study of the body composition, nutrition, and health of military women and will be making recommendations.

Vaccines and Prophylactic Treatment

The military has had long experience with vaccine administration. Seven vaccines (oral polio vaccine, diphtheria-tetanus, adenovirus 4 and 7, meningococcus A, CYWI35, influenza, and measles-rubella) are administered to Army recruits during basic training. Seven other vaccines (hepatitis B, hepatitis A, yellow fever, Japanese encephalitis, plague, rabies, and cholera) are given for deployment to high-risk areas, to alert forces as required by a host country, or as directed by the surgeon general. Each of these vaccines can produce local or systemic reactions in recipients. The "antigenic load" injected into service members is considerable, which has raised questions about possible unhealthy long-term effects. However, no known adverse long-term effects of standard immunization have been identified in PGW military personnel.

The threat of CBW and questions regarding exposures to CBW agents have been raised as issues in assessing adverse health consequences of service in the PG. Reports from U.S. government agencies and United Nations (UN) sources (UN, 1995) indicated that the Iraqi forces had experimental chemical and biological weapons programs and also had both biological and chemical munitions available for use in the field. The list of agents reported by the UN special commission to have been in the Iraqi program includes chemical agents such as sulfur mustard, sarin, and VX and biological agents such as botulinus toxin, anthrax, aflatoxin, ricin, mycotoxins, hemorrhagic conjunctivitis virus, rotavirus, and wheat cover smut.

Multiple reports of the detection of chemical agents during ODS were received and investigated by U.S. military and intelligence agencies. The conclusions of several independent investigative and advisory bodies have been that there is no credible evidence that chemical or biological weapons were used by Iraq in the PGW (DSB, 1994; IOM, 1995a; NIH Technology Assessment Workshop Panel, 1994). It is not clear, however, whether various statements about this matter refer to combat use, other military use, accidental or inadvertent exposure, or something else. Serious concerns among veterans and some investigators persist that significant exposure to these agents may have occurred, specifically in noncombat situations, and the possibility of exposure is being evaluated by the President's Advisory Committee (PAC) on Persian Gulf Veterans' Illnesses and the PGW Veterans' Illnesses Investigation Team (PGVIIT).

At the time this report was completed, the committee had not learned of any reports of confirmed troop exposures to CBW agents. However, as this report was being peer-reviewed, the committee learned, in June 1996, from press coverage and congressional testimony (Joseph, 1996), that troops located near an Iraqi munitions bunker that was destroyed in early March 1991 may have been exposed to low levels of chemical agent. This information was also outlined in a letter the committee received in July 1996 from the office of the director of central intelligence, in response to a letter sent in May 1996 by the committee chair requesting information on the current knowledge of possible chemical exposures. The response also indicated that work was being done in conjunction with the DoD PGVIIT to "resolve whether some U.S. personnel could have been exposed to chemical agent" (Landry, 1996). Also, the description of one sulfur mustard contact that occurred in a bunker has been designated unconfirmed by DoD (Dunn, 1996), and two incidents reported earlier by the Czechs have recently been classified as credible (PAC, 1996d; PGVIIT, 1996).

Recent attention has been given to the possibility that the bombing and destruction of Iraqi CBW facilities may have led to the atmospheric dispersion of sarin or possibly other CBW agents (PAC, 1996b,c). Representatives of the Central Intelligence Agency (CIA) testified to the PAC that any possible release of toxic agents from the destruction of these facilities would not have resulted in exposure of U.S. troops, since atmospheric modeling of the conditions present at the time of the relevant bombing suggests that any cloud generated by explosives would move away from coalition forces (PAC, 1996b). Others have suggested, however, the possibility that agents such as sarin were deposited into the upper atmosphere and fell on coalition troops within the last weeks of the air war (Tuite, 1996).

The results of atmospheric models applied to possible production of low levels of agents of any kind from bombing destruction were not available for review by the committee. Finally, there is no available evidence in human or animal studies to date that exposure to nerve agents at low levels that do not produce any detectable acute clinical or physiological manifestations results in any chronic or long-term adverse health effects. The recent evidence that destruction of a storage bunker could have resulted in the release of a small amount of nerve agent has to be explored. Specifically, the committee believes that animal research and human epidemiologic studies should be conducted to determine whether long-term neurotoxic effects of low-level exposures to nerve agents can be observed.

In evaluating the possibility that CBW agents affected the health of veterans, the committee relied heavily on known toxicological and pathological effects and existing knowledge regarding short- and long-term health effects of CBW agents and on findings reported from extensive DoD and DVA clinical evaluations of veterans. To date, there are no confirmed reports of clinical manifestations of acute nerve agent exposure. Further work, which has been proposed by DoD, should be completed as rapidly as is feasible.

Threats of possible biological warfare use were reported as troops were deployed. Because of concern that the Iraqi forces could use biological agents against U.S. personnel during ODS, vaccines were made available to selected groups. DoD vaccinated some troops against anthrax and some against botulism, which were considered the biological warfare agents most likely to be encountered. Anthrax vaccine was widely used. Botulinum toxoid was given to a much smaller number of marines and soldiers. Individuals receiving botulinum toxin vaccine were supposed to sign a list to indicate their consent.

Several factors have created questions about these vaccines. Although each vaccine was intended to prevent serious disease induced by these potential biological weapons, they were unique in the military immunization program and were administered in the field after deployment. Because the vaccination program was classified as secret, some concern has been raised as to whether vaccines were administered without consent or without appropriate approvals from the Food and Drug Administration (FDA). These concerns have raised further questions about a possible role of these vaccines in the long-term health effects reported by some recipients. The interim PAC report presents a good discussion of the issues surrounding vaccine administration (PAC, 1996a).

The anthrax vaccination program was involuntary; the vaccine is approved for general use and did not require consent for administration. The recommended dosage schedule of anthrax vaccine for laboratory workers is six injections over an 18-month period. Few service members in ODS received more than the first two doses, given 2 weeks apart. The program was discontinued when the war was over. It is estimated that about 150,000 service members received at least one dose. The known side effects of the vaccine include tenderness, erythema, and swelling at the injection site in about 6% of recipients. Less that 1% have more severe local reactions, which may limit the use of the arm for 1–2 days. Reaction rates among those receiving the vaccine in ODS were unmeasured, although one person was hospitalized because of an infection at the injection site.

Botulinum toxoid vaccine consists of five of the most common types of toxins (A, B, C, D, E) that have been converted to toxoid by use of formalin, with alum as an adjuvant. Botulinum toxoid vaccine has the status of an investigational product with FDA and has been used as an investigational vaccine to protect high-risk laboratory workers for more than 20 years. Reaction rates have been estimated after administration of the vaccine at USAMRIID as follows: mild local reactions have been more frequent (up to 10%) than with anthrax vaccine; about 3% experienced mild systemic reactions such as headache, myalgia, fever, and malaise for 48–72 hours. No chronic sequelae have been reported.

The vaccine is to be given in three injections: an initial dose, followed by other injections at 2 and 12 weeks, with a booster at 1 year. About 8,000 service members received at least one dose. U.S. recipients of the botulinum toxoid vaccine were primarily members of the First Marine Division and the Army VII Corps. All members of these units were to have had the opportunity to volunteer and to give informed consent before receiving the vaccine. Reaction data were not collected.

As of this writing, DoD indicated that the validated reconstruction of some PGW immunization records had been entered into the Comprehensive Clinical Evaluation Program (CCEP) database, including 5,190 Army anthrax records (of a total of approximately 150,000 recipients), 3,875 Navy or Marine (1 Army) botulinum toxoid records (of a total of approximately 8,000 recipients), and 204 Army records of those receiving both anthrax and botulinum toxoid vaccines. These data have also been given to those working with the GIS at USACHPPM, to add to the exposure database under development.

Pyridostigmine Bromide

PB belongs to the group of drugs classified as anticholinergic that bind reversibly with acetylcholinesterase (AChE), an enzyme essential to the metabolism of acetylcholine. PB and related drugs allow the temporary buildup of acetylcholine, which causes continuous stimulation of cholinergic receptors throughout the central and peripheral nervous systems. This pharmacological action would be useful in protecting military personnel from the effects of certain chemical warfare agents (organophosphate nerve agents) that bind irreversibly with AChE and can cause lethal and life-threatening complications. PB competes for binding sites and allows escape of some AChE to permit more controlled transmission of nerve impulses. Anti-AChE agents are not new drugs. The first drug in this group, physostigmine, was developed in 1864. PB has been used for decades at doses of 360–6,000 mg daily to treat patients with a neuromuscular disease called myasthenia gravis. There is a great deal of pharmacological and clinical data, therefore, on the use of PB and related drugs.

Anti-AChE agents can worsen certain medical conditions, including asthma, coronary artery disease, and cardiac dysrhythmias (especially bradycardia). Persons who are sensitive to PB may develop anaphylactic shock. These conditions occur promptly after a dose or an overdose; discontinuation of the drug and administration of atropine lead to rapid recovery in most people. DoD has been criticized for insufficient study of this compound before its use to protect military personnel in the war against Iraq, even though PB was used in a dosage of 30 mg given three times a day, lower than that approved for use in patients with myasthenia gravis. Troops were given a 1-week supply of the pills, to be taken at the direction of the commanding officer. Although this was the recommended dose, it is not known how much was actually taken.

Previously reported side effects of PB use in patient populations, generally at higher doses, include those expected from stimulation of the peripheral parasympathetic nervous system, including nausea, vomiting, diarrhea, abdominal cramps, increased peristalsis, increased salivation, bronchial secretions, miosis, and diaphoresis. Neuromuscular junctions in skeletal muscle are also stimulated; the effects include muscle cramps, fasciculation, and weakness. The bromide radical can cause skin rashes that usually subside when the drug is stopped. There have been no documented long-term side effects of PB. Use of PB has not been contraindicated during pregnancy. All of the side effects noted above were reported in PG military personnel taking PB for various periods. Gastrointestinal symptoms were the most common complaint.

One study failed to show any significant difference in symptoms in small numbers of volunteers taking PB versus a placebo in a desert environment (Cook et al., 1992). PB does raise body temperature slightly because it decreases blood flow to the skin, thus limiting heat loss by convection. Offsetting this effect is the increased sweating caused by PB. In the volunteer study, the slight increase in temperature did not affect exercise tolerance in a heated chamber.

Since the PGW, DoD has examined the safety, tolerance, pharmacokinetics, and pharmacodynamics of PB in a double-blind evaluation of 90 male and female volunteers. The same dose was assessed (30 mg given every 8 hours for 21 days) as used by troops during ODS/S. Analysis of the data showed that the drug was safe and well tolerated. There were no differences between the active drug group and the placebo group in the frequency of mild adverse effects such as headache, dizziness, nausea, hypotension, rash, and alopecia. There were no chronic effects after a year of follow-up. The muscarinic action of the drug caused self-limiting gastrointestinal complaints in four persons. Multiple lab tests were not affected. Special emphasis on hormone analyses demonstrated a few changes, but these were determined to be biologically insignificant. Thus, the ingestion of PB in these adults did not result in unexpected side effects or pharmacological activity (Lasseter and Garg, 1996).

Some explanations for a high incidence of symptoms after PB ingestion have been suggested. First, the reactions of women may differ from those of men, especially if women are taking birth control pills; the effects of PB on women had not been studied prior to the PGW. Second, the troops were not screened for those conditions that are contraindications to use of PB, including asthma, peptic ulcer, liver disease, kidney disease, or hypersensitivity to PB, although predeployment medical examinations generally should ensure that these conditions (other than hypersensitivity) were present in few of the troops on active duty. A third hypothesis is that there were synergistic reactions among some combination of PB, pesticides, and insect repellents used by the troops. It has been known for many years that the simultaneous or sequential administration of two anti-AChE drugs can have an additive or even a synergistic effect. Robbins and Cherniack (1986) have reported that Deet (an insect repellent widely used during the PGW) is only partially absorbed through the skin of humans and is rapidly but not completely excreted. Deet impairs mammalian biochemical pathways (reversibly inhibiting the urea cycle) and can block lactate-dependent synthesis of glucose (Brini and Tremblay, 1991; Heick et al., 1988).

Interactions of Exposures

Pesticides such as permethrin (i.e., synthetic pyrethroids) modify the ionic permeability of nerve membranes and produce a neuroexcitatory toxic response

(Casida et al., 1983; Vijverberg and van den Bercken, 1990). They have been shown to act on sodium channels in nerve membranes in a fashion directly dependent on the structural conformation of the pesticides (Eells et al., 1992). Permethrin has also been found to inhibit calcium-dependent ATPase (adenosine triphosphatase) enzyme activity in cells from the central nervous system (Kodavanti et al., 1993).

One investigator has suggested that the interaction or coexposure of chickens to PB, Deet, and permethrin is associated with significantly greater neurotoxicity than that induced by exposure to one agent alone. Abou-Donia et al. (1996) have reported that concurrent administration of these compounds to chickens causes markedly greater neurotoxicity than that resulting from treatment with any individual compound. The investigators also note that there is a known polymorphism in the butylcholinesterase enzyme that could further exacerbate the demonstrated interaction of these compounds.

The investigators point out that the actual exposure conditions present in the PG are not mimicked by the doses administered in the chicken experiments because the experimental doses and routes of administration were not directly comparable to use by troops in the PG. In addition, it is not clear that a significant number of participants in the PGW were exposed to all three of these compounds simultaneously. The investigators note that polymorphisms described in the genes that code for cholinesterases could exacerbate the interactions they observed when similar exposures are encountered in humans (McGuire et al., 1989). They also note a recent study reporting that individuals who are homozygous for the rare variant allele of the butylcholinesterase gene may be at above-average risk of cholinergic side effects from pyridostigmine. While these reported findings have been challenged as not representative of the human in vivo situation (Lotti and Moretto, 1995), they may have some relevance for acute effects from pyridostigmine administration. The committee is not aware of data suggesting that chronic health effects are associated with this type of short-term enzyme inhibition. It is conceivable that increased severity of clinical signs and symptoms after coexposure to these compounds is related to their effects on the target proteins in the nervous system.

Other recent data illustrate how the interaction of environmental compounds can synergistically enhance receptor-mediated responses. Arnold et al. (1996) have used a yeast-based system that incorporates the human estrogen receptor to test the estrogenic activity of environmental compounds used alone and in combination, specifically asking whether the compounds interact to enhance estrogenic potency. They studied compounds such as pesticides and various polychlorinated agents and demonstrated that these environmental contaminants can synergistically enhance normal estrogenic activity. This work raises new questions about the mechanisms of action of steroid hormones such as estrogen. Further, it provides new insight into the complex interplay of environmental signals with receptor-mediated biological responses. It is not clear whether this work has implications for the health of persons exposed to complex environmental agents. However, it does illustrate the need for continued research into the basic biology of interaction of multiple toxins and the normal cellular response.

Molecular epidemiologic investigation of possible gene–environment interactions in the production of adverse health outcomes related to cholinergic overstimulation could be informative. The committee recommends that such research be carried out after careful consideration of the relevant hypothesis and peer review of the proposed protocol. With the lack of a defined case for studying unexplained illnesses and with little evidence that chronic health effects are seen from pyridostigmine, the precise path for investigators to follow in the study of PGW veterans remains to be clarified.

Other medications could possibly increase the risk of side effects of PB. Simultaneous use of PB and a β-blocker such as those used to treat hypertension could cause a further reduction in cardiac output and blood pressure. In rare cases, there could be bronchial constriction. A combination of PB with medications that cause vasodilation (e.g., calcium channel blockers or direct-acting vasodilators) in circumstances of poor hydration could lead to light-headed feelings or syncope. Antimalarial medications in combination with PB could lead to diarrhea. Quinidine and PB combined could induce heart block, but the former is not used routinely for malaria prophylaxis or treatment. All of these possible drug interactions (and others not mentioned) cause acute and short-term problems. The committee knows of no evidence of any chronic effect.

Depleted Uranium

DU is used by DoD in antitank munitions and in tank armor because of its very high density and pyrophoric properties; in other words, it can punch through very heavy armor and it burns fiercely. DU is a by-product of the process that removes much of the potent and highly radioactive isotopes U-238 and U-235, as well as U-234, from uranium. DU typically contains only 0.2% U-235 and 0.001% U-234, and its radioactivity is approximately 50% that of natural uranium (Daxon, 1994).

The major toxicity of DU is from its chemical rather than its radioactive properties. For instance, DU has the potential to cause kidney damage (Daxon and Musk, 1993). Irreparable kidney damage has been shown in studies of injected or inhaled uranium salts. For acute exposures, kidney toxicity results from 1–3 μg of uranium per gram of kidney (Diamond, 1989). However, there is considerable uncertainly regarding the toxicity of long-term exposure to uranium (Crawford-Brown and Wilson, 1984).

Radiation exposure from intact DU munitions and armor is minimal and within accepted standards. A series of studies conducted by DoD measured the radiation exposure received by personnel during the transportation, storage, and use of DU-containing systems. Studies have shown that with the exception of warehouses in which large quantities of DU munitions were stored, the estimated annual exposure did not exceed the current standard of 100 mrem/year for the general population (GAO, 1993a). Where this limit might be exceeded, standard radiation protection programs were in place (Daxon, 1994).

The radiological and toxicological hazards associated with long-term exposure to imbedded fragments are uncertain. There are no known studies of the long-term effects of DU metal implanted in tissues. Few ODS/S personnel were exposed to DU. Activities of the 144th Service and Supply Company in fighting fires, recovering vehicles, and cleaning the 29 tanks damaged by DU munitions led to the potential exposure of 27 soldiers. Results from testing 12 of these soldiers were reported as negative (GAO, 1993a), and the remaining 15 soldiers chose not to be tested (DSB, 1994). It is possible that there was wider exposure to DU of troops who entered destroyed enemy vehicles either on duty or as sightseers or of combat-support troops who were exposed to battle dust after tank battles or to contaminated smoke from explosion and fire in the destruction of ammunition storage.

A friendly fire incident wounded approximately 35 U.S. soldiers, of whom approximately 22 were suspected to have retained DU fragments (Daxon, 1993). These wounded soldiers were offered close follow-up after the war as part of a DVA-funded medical surveillance program. Thirty-three of these 35 soldiers continue to be followed and studied. After 3 years, 15 of the 33 soldiers had detectable shrapnel. The initial work has demonstrated no evidence of toxicologic effects, but it has been noted that uranium excretion is significantly higher in soldiers with known retained shrapnel, supporting the contention that the shrapnel is not inert (Keogh, 1995).

Currently, two animal studies funded by DoD are under way to evaluate the long-term effects of DU. The first study is designed to investigate a rodent model of DU tumorigenesis and is being conducted by investigators at the Armed Forces Radiation Research Institute. Since little is known of the precise tumorigenic potential of this material, these researchers propose to conduct a long-term study in male F344 rats. The protocol includes a low- and high-dose 2- to 3-year exposure to implanted natural uranium wires. At the same time a companion study of the renal toxicity of DU is also proposed. This study will investigate the kinetics of renal excretion of uranium and possible toxicity from long-term exposure.

These studies are useful in that they provide additional information about the chronic toxicity of uranium compounds. However, since the investigators must use nondepleted uranium and since available data indicate that the carcinogenicity of this compound is likely to be low, it is not known whether these experiments will add important new information.

The second study, conducted at the Inhalation Toxicology Research Institute, is a 3-year rodent study utilizing three doses of DU with implanted tantalum and nonimplanted sham controls to study the behavioral effects of DU and the histologic and biochemical effects of implanted exposure and to evaluate uranium distribution throughout the body. CNS effects of exposure will be studied by evaluation of autonomic, sensorimotor, and neuromuscular alterations. Excitability and arousal also will be measured. Peripheral nerve conduction will be measured and hippocampal electrophysiology will be studied. Blood and urine samples will be collected and chemistries done. The bones (femur), hippocampus, sciatic nerve, kidney, liver, spleen, and muscles will be studied histologically. Renal function will be examined in detail. Finally, the tissue distribution of uranium will be quantified.

This protocol will provide detailed information on the toxicity of DU in rodents, which is useful information. However, studies already completed suggest that there is little evidence that DU will produce any novel toxic picture.

PSYCHOSOCIAL EXPOSURES

A wide array of potentially toxic environmental agents has been considered in relation to health and ODS/S service. These include not only physical and chemical hazards but also the personal, social, and organizational context of service in the Gulf, the stressors present or generated in each domain, and the effects of these stressors on service personnel. Both physiological and psychological stress responses occur when humans are confronted with demands to adapt, change, or reorganize their lives or ways of thinking about themselves and those about them (Stretch et al., 1996). Stressors are those events or circumstances that produce challenge or threat.

It is not easy to compare the levels of stress, or the responses to stress, in the PGW with those in previous military engagements. One difference is that PG military personnel did not have the level of detachment possible in prior conflicts. Easy telephone communication to family and friends, up-to-date news services, even the very rapid mobilization itself tended to keep people's "heads" back home while their bodies were in the Gulf theater. Another difference was that some of the accustomed ways of relieving stress were simply absent, among them interchange with the indigenous population (almost entirely forbidden) and access to alcoholic beverages (also forbidden). Further, the stress was acute, and it was everywhere, even far from the front lines. Entry into that situation was rapid, with little opportunity to prepare or be prepared. Similarly, reentry into U.S. society was rapid, with very little time or opportunity to accommodate.

A further difference of the PGW from most earlier conflicts is that U.S. combat troops in the PG experienced very low levels of casualties and benefited from vastly improved means of dealing with infectious diseases. Puzzling reactions and symptoms seen during and after prior conflicts may have been incorrectly attributed to battle casualties and infectious diseases that were considered unavoidable and even relatively acceptable outcomes of war. Thus, the lower prevalence of battle injuries and infections in the Gulf theater may have unmasked psychophysiological symptoms that were present in earlier conflicts but attributed to injury and casualty.

The individual's perception and appraisal of events play a strong role in shaping the impact of stress. Most personnel who served in the PG would probably concur that the constant threat of CBW was stressful, that SCUD attacks and uncertain risk of other attacks or counterattacks by the Iraqi army were stressful, and that field conditions were often stressful. At the same time, each individual perceived the specific events associated with his or her experience in the PGW as more or less stressful. Moreover, events in the theater were experienced in the context of life situations predating the PGW, and the novel stressors of deployment were superimposed on the unique physical, physiologic, and mental state of each person.

In anticipation of the psychological stress that would be created by a high-threat deployment to a harsh environment for ODS/S, DoD initiated a series of studies of the stress of deployment by sending a research team to SWA during September 1990 as the theater was being established. Beginning with that initial study, a 2-year program of studies after ODS/S has been conducted under the leadership of Dr. David Marlowe, Chief, Department of Military Psychiatry, Walter Reed Army Institute of Research (WRAIR). This program has focused on the stresses and psychological consequences of ODS/S and, more recently, has addressed symptoms experienced by the troops.

This program has gathered data describing the stressors associated with ODS/S deployment from a variety of sources, as follows:

1. data collected before combat from active army in SWA (approximately 1,200 persons in individual and group interviews, plus 2,850 by questionnaire);
2. data collected after combat, time 1 (approximately 800 persons in individual and group interviews, plus 9,800 deployers and 830 controls by questionnaire);
3. data collected after combat, time 2 (4,585 deployers and 2,249 controls by questionnaire);
4. data collected from Pennsylvania and Hawaii, 2 years after combat (1,739 deployed and 2,512 not deployed by questionnaire); and
5. additional data collected 2 years after combat from U.S. Army National Guard and U.S. Army reserve troops (1,420 deployed to SWA and 1,995 not deployed) and U.S. Army Individual Ready Reserves (IRR) (500 deployed to SWA and 695 not deployed to SWA by questionnaire).

These studies are discussed in sequence below. Studies of active duty units included men only; studies with reserve units included men and 8–9% women (Marlowe, 1996).

Stressors Associated with Deployment

Studies of stress experienced by PGW veterans deployed prior to the beginning of the ground war were conducted during September and October 1990 (Marlowe et al., 1990a) and during November and December 1990 (Marlowe et al., 1990b); major findings are presented. Active Army members participated in individual or small-group interviews with others of the same rank. The purposes of these studies were to determine how stressful the deployment was and the sustainability over time of the force in the theater. The most consistently reported source of stress during this period was lack of knowledge of probable tour length and return date, as well as lack of knowledge of whether the troops would be called on for a protracted siege or combat—in other words, uncertainty about the parameters of deployment.

Examples of other stressors for some persons or groups in the theater include separation from family and concerns about home; difficulties with mail or telephone communications with home; heavy workload and sleep deprivation, especially for combat support and service units; unsatisfactory living conditions, including extreme crowding with resultant interpersonal pressure and hostility; apprehensions about being in imminent danger; social and psychological isolation of members of combat arms units; leadership issues including poor morale; the lack of recreation facilities; heat, sand, and the desert environment; and the severity of climatic conditions. Once telecommunications were in place, soldiers could benefit from communicating with their families at home, which remained a primary source of support (Wright et al., 1991).

Major contributors to the stresses of ODS deployment included the high estimation of Iraqi military capabilities and media anticipation of very high casualties, the threat of CBW with related fears about the adequacy of MOPP (mission objective protective posture) gear, and concerns about terrorism and infiltration. For support troops, particularly those arriving later in the theater, there was increasing apprehension about Iraqi capacities and the effectiveness of U.S. gear. Confusion about and multiple changes in deployment departure dates were also contributing factors (Marlowe, 1995).

Anticipation of Combat

As conditions in the theater matured, access to amenities improved, deprivation decreased, and events became more focused. Soldiers began to experience more stress related to the anticipation of combat. The most salient of these anticipated stressors were having a buddy killed, attack by enemy aircraft, attack by enemy tanks, being wounded or killed, attack by enemy artillery, CBW attack, and inadequate medical care. The most prevalent of these were chemical or biological attack (65%) and having a buddy killed (55%) (Marlowe, 1995). Confusion about media estimates of potential casualty rates was a major concern for those in combat units, whereas concern about failure of weapons systems at critical points in the event of combat was more evident among support units (Wright et al., 1991).

It was evident to researchers at this early time that deployment was more disruptive for reservists and their families than for active duty service members. Unexpected, relatively sudden changes in circumstances created significant financial and job-related concerns for many reasons. The ODS experience of support units, many of whom were reservists, also differed from that of combat units, most of whom were on active duty. Many support units had heavier workloads, crowded and primitive living arrangements, and less clearly defined roles and missions (Wright et al., 1991).

Time spent in SWA prior to the initiation of war increased stress, probably because of the stringent conditions of deployment for combat arms troops. Anticipation of combat was stressful, but commencement of the ground war actually relieved the stress that had built up over months of anticipation (WRAIR, 1992).

Combat Exposure

Major fears during the initial assault were of CBW, augmented by conflicting information about the effective life of MOPP gear and conflicting beliefs about the effects of antichemical and antibiological medications. As many as 40% of soldiers in all units studied experienced incoming indirect fire; 40% of one unit and 70% of another reported experiencing mines and booby traps; 40% in two units claimed to have fired rounds at the enemy and 30% to have engaged in a firefight; about 18% in two units claimed a confirmed "kill"; about 80% in one unit and 60% in another saw enemy killed or wounded in action; and about 44% in one unit and 36% in another saw civilians killed or wounded in action (WRAIR, 1992). Less than 2% of the soldiers in all three brigades were injured or wounded themselves. About 14% in two units reported seeing an American soldier wounded; fewer reported seeing an American soldier killed. More than 10% reported a buddy wounded or injured. About 25% in one brigade, and 8 and 10% in two others, reported seeing an American wounded by friendly fire; 1–3% of persons in these units indicated they had seen an American killed. More than 20% in two units felt at some point that they were in imminent danger of being killed (WRAIR, 1992). Although actual casualty rates were low, perceptions of danger were widespread due to fears of CBW. The most stressful events were those involving lethality or injury. The greatest combat trauma was in circumstances of "intimate violence" (e.g., vehicles in which a crew member was killed or wounded). Friendly fire had the greatest emotional impact when it involved parties from the same company or battalion. There were few combat stress casualties requiring intervention in the field (WRAIR, 1992).

Additional factors that some troops identified as stressful during postcombat debriefings included having to take "untried experimental" drugs and vaccines (PB, anthrax vaccine) with rumored "terrible" side effects, continued attacks on civilians by Iraqis, oil fires and smoke, concern about time of return home, accidental losses of unit members, concern about family and family adjustment on return, and memories of traumatic events (Marlowe, 1995).

Aftermath and Long-Term Adjustment

Stress related to combat was only one of several categories of stressors affecting soldiers after their return home from ODS. Stressors that were part of the aftermath of combat experienced by the VIIth Corps 6–12 months after ODS included the following in descending order of significance: unit/workplace climate, ODS-related stressors, reassignment and movement, downsizing of military, and family issues (Marlowe, 1995). ODS-related stressors include concerns with ODS experiences in the field and problems after return from the theater.

Two years after return from ODS, four intercurrent stress factors, in descending order of significance, were reported by members of the XVIIIth Corps as follows: ODS-related issues, health and finances, unit climate, and downsizing or job future issues (Marlowe, 1995). Although major sources of stress 1 and 2 years after ODS were related to current life issues for most soldiers, a significant subgroup still saw their life problems as arising out of ODS/S experiences (Marlowe, 1995).

During 1993, at the request of Congress, DoD conducted additional studies of veterans in Pennsylvania and Hawaii. A total sample of 4,334 veterans responding to a survey was studied (31% response rate): 1,739 were deployed during ODS/S (1,524 to the PG and 215 to other locations), 2,512 were not deployed, and 83 had an unknown deployment status. There were 715 active duty soldiers and 766 reservists among the deployed and 1,576 active duty troops and 948 reservists among the nondeployed (Stretch et al., 1995, 1996). Although the response rate is low, opening the possibility of bias in the findings, the general orders of magnitude of the stressors may be reliable.

Stressor clusters of deployment identified retrospectively in the Pennsylvania and Hawaii study by reservists included possible exposure to traumatic events, actual exposure to traumatic events, stresses of waiting for deployment, stresses in the theater, and stresses at home. The pattern of stressors was similar for the active duty component, with the exception of their exposure to explicit stressors of combat such as being fired on by the enemy and engaging the enemy in firefights. Exposure to oil fires and concern about that exposure also have been stressors. Two years after the end of ODS/S, 50% of those who claimed exposure to oil well fires had at least moderate concern over that exposure (USAMRMC, 1994).

When asked to rate their current stress levels (two years after ODS), 66 and 67% of the active duty and reserve study participants who were deployed said they were experiencing moderate to extreme stress compared with 59 and 55% of the nondeployed active duty and reserve troops. When asked about the effects of stress on their lives, 46 and 41% of the active duty and reserve troops who were deployed responded that the effects were moderate or greater, compared with 35 and 30%, respectively, of the nondeployed (USAMRMC, 1994).

In sum, "deployment of American forces to SWA created an interacting nexus of acute, subacute, and enduring chronic stressors and stress responses" (USAMRMC, 1994). Troops had been prepared for prolonged imminent danger from combat and simultaneously had to deal with a variety of other war-related changes, including a demanding workload.

Stressors identified in DoD studies were also indicated in DVA studies. Reserve troops studied after they returned from ODS/S ($N = 215$) by Sutker et al. (1993) identified (as stressful) separation from home, family, and friends (18%); SCUD missile attacks (15%); austere physical environment (13%); loss of control, uncertainty, and fear of the unknown (8%); lack of leadership (7%); protracted delays in return home after hostilities (5%); inadequate supplies and equipment (5%); prolonged truck transport in the desert (4%); lack of information (4%); and financial difficulties (3%). These findings were borne out by Wolfe et al. (1992c, 1993) in studies of the Fort Devens Reunion Survey.

Concerns that existing scales to assess war stress are not sensitive to experiences of women, ethnically diverse groups, or married and older military personnel (a rapidly growing segment of the volunteer-based U.S. forces) prompted Wolfe et al. (1993) to assess 2,344 PGW veterans (including 208 women) to investigate the following three major stressor categories: traditional wartime activities, nontraditional wartime events, and non–war zone deployment-related experiences (domestic, vocational, and psychosocial stressors). Veterans returning through Fort Devens, Massachusetts (including active duty personnel, reservists, and National Guard men and women), were evaluated within 5 days of their return from ODS/S and before they rejoined their families. Stressors predictive of posttraumatic stress disorder (PTSD) were measured by the Lauffer combat exposure scale score, a checklist expanded to reflect ODS war zone experiences, and an open-ended format where respondents described the most distressing incident of their deployment (Wolfe et al., 1993). These same stressors were associated with Mississippi Scale scores (PTSD) and Brief Symptom Inventory (BSI)/General Severity Index (GSI) scores indicating general psychological distress (Wolfe et al., 1993). Sutker et al. (1993) found that high levels of war zone stress, estimated by the ODS war zone stress exposure scale (developed by J. Wolfe and described earlier) were associated with greater numbers of psychological symptoms, negative moods, PTSD symptoms, and physical or somatic symptoms among 215 veterans evaluated in New Orleans.

Sutker et al. (1994a,b) also evaluated the influence of particularly gruesome war zone trauma in studies of troops mobilized to the PG for graves registration duty. This duty involved handling the dead, as well as mutilated body parts (e.g., matching body parts to the remainder of a corpse). Among 24 personnel studied, 46% met criteria for PTSD. This study was replicated with a larger sample ($N = 60$) of reservists who had been activated for service. Among those who were deployed to the PG, 48% had a current diagnosis of PTSD and 65% had PTSD in their lifetime. Among those who were not deployed there were no reports of current or lifetime PTSD (Sutker et al., 1994b). These DVA-sponsored studies have contributed uniquely to understanding the stressors related to the transition home from the theater, and the data may be useful in planning support for troops (especially reservists) in the future.

Gender Differences in Exposure to Stress

Women's health problems may be linked not only to their experiences with the declared enemy in the PGW but also to actions by U.S. troops (e.g., sexual harassment or assault). Sexual harassment and assault during deployment created social and physical stressors that may cause symptoms in the years after the PGW (Wolfe et al., 1992b).

Sexual assault and harassment were studied among 142 women reservists who served in the Gulf and responded to a questionnaire 1 year after return. These women were a self-selected sample of a larger group of 241 women originally studied by Wolfe. Of the participants, 8% reported attempted or completed sexual assault, 31% reported physical harassment, and 63% reported verbal harassment during their Gulf War deployment (Wolfe et al., 1992b).

Issues raised regarding some additional stressors for women included gender discrimination and low supplies of feminine sanitary products. Concerns for privacy, important to both men and women, become particularly crucial when men and women serve together in close proximity, as they did in the Gulf.

Studies currently under way are examining further the effects of stress from harassment among women. In addition to studies of sexual harassment, this committee supports the recommendations of another IOM committee that recently reported in detail on research needs resulting from military women and men living and working together in close quarters, in addition to those related to sexual harassment, including the following (IOM, 1995b):

- the extent and impact of sex-role stereotyping of military women by military officers, noncommissioned officers, and enlisted personnel;

- the prevalence, contributing factors, and effect of physical and sexual assaults and sexual harassment of women in the Armed Forces;
- effects of premilitary sexual abuse or violence history and military traumatic experiences on psychological health and job performance;
- outcomes of treatment for traumatized servicewomen; and
- strategies for handling sanitary needs.

DVA ENVIRONMENTAL HAZARDS RESEARCH CENTERS

In January 1994, DVA announced a program to establish centers for basic and clinical science studies of environmental hazards. Up to $500,000 per year for 5 years would be provided for support of the centers to engage in basic research on environmental health effects, with special emphasis on the diagnosis and treatment of medical problems currently being reported by PGW veterans. The DVA was especially interested in new initiatives that complemented current activities and suggested that interorganizational agreements and scientific affiliations be encouraged, if they were justified and properly set up; this would include collaboration with non-DVA researchers.

The environmental hazards research centers (EHRCs) were established in July 1994 in the DVA Medical Centers (VAMCs) in Boston, Massachusetts; East Orange, New Jersey; and Portland, Oregon. The environmental centers were fully funded by the end of 1994.

The committee received written materials and heard oral presentations by representatives from each of the DVA EHRCs. Overall, the research activities, selected for funding by the DVA Central Office, are investigator-initiated, reflect local interests and expertise, and will have some serious limitations in broader use for either understanding causes of illness in returning PG veterans or assisting in determining whether returning veterans had illnesses different from or more frequent than might have occurred had these persons not been deployed. It is unclear whether or how these funded research activities are being managed by any research coordinating body of either DoD or DVA. The committee learned, as this report was being finalized, that the centers were reviewed on-site in March 1996 by external reviewers and that comments and responses by the EHRCs will be reviewed by the Research Working Group (RWG) of the PG Veterans Coordinating Board.

Research at the Portland EHRC is focused on unexpected illnesses as reported by returning PG veterans, with a particular focus on threats to the neurologic and musculoskeletal systems (reflecting complaints reported by veterans with symptoms but without diagnoses). As is true elsewhere, few data documenting actual exposures are available. Temporal segments of activity (Operation Desert Shield only, Operation Desert Storm only, desert cleanup only, etc.) are highly inaccurate surrogates for exposures and create the potential for unknown heterogeneity and misclassification. A majority of Portland's respondents to date have not elected to join the DVA PG Health Registry (PGHR), further emphasizing that the PGHR is not an appropriate tool for research. Use of sophisticated neuroendocrine tests performed many years after the conflict can have only limited usefulness in characterizing risks of deployment or reentry after the conflict.

Researchers at the East Orange, New Jersey, EHRC hypothesize that chronic fatigue and chemical sensitivity are associated with many of the unexplained symptoms and illnesses among returning PG veterans. Criteria for chronic fatigue syndrome (CFS) changed from those proposed in 1988 to less restrictive criteria in 1994. The syndrome is poorly characterized and not universally accepted as valid. If chronic fatigue and chemical sensitivity become accepted medical entities, the lack of population-based estimates of frequency and severity will still complicate assessment of whether these syndromes among returning veterans are associated with or caused by military service. The use of extensive (and expensive) laboratory tests of immune function, interferons, and cytokines and the numerous magnetic resonance imagings (MRIs) of these people raise questions about resource allocation. Developing objective measures of the effects of chemical exposures on possibly chemically sensitive individuals has been proposed as one of the center projects and may be of some utility in civilian settings, but it will have little practical application in the mobilization and deployment of large numbers of healthy troops unless future epidemiologic work, utilizing accepted diagnostic criteria, demonstrates an increased prevalence among deployed veterans. Such measures might then be used as premobilization screening to assist in later diagnostic evaluation of symptomatic individuals. The project that hypothesizes individual differences in susceptibility to stress and vulnerability is intriguing, although the challenges of interspecies extrapolation from rodent models will require careful interpretation.

Studies at the Boston EHRC will, in part, continue to utilize the longitudinal follow-up of a group of PG veterans who returned through Fort Devens, Massachusetts. Although this appears to be a strength, the small number of participants is likely to limit investigators' abilities to address their research questions. Clinical studies of the hypotheses that higher exposures to combustion products of oil well fires impair pulmonary function 5 years or more after exposure are unlikely to be fruitful, in part because of the small sample size. A state-specific study (Massachusetts) of differential cancer incidence among returnees may have too few events to justify support, particularly given the young age of most of the deployed force. If this were to be judged as an important undertaking, a larger group—perhaps even the entire cohort of approximately 697,000 returning veterans—could better address such questions of cancer incidence and mortality.

In summary, the DVA-funded EHRCs facilitate the application of research skills available at selected VAMCs across the United States, but these research efforts will have limited ability, individually or collectively, to contribute to understanding the health effects of military service in the PGW. The committee has not evaluated other uses of these research programs.

4

Health Outcomes

OVERVIEW

This chapter reviews the empirical evidence available to the committee through May 1996 regarding the health experience of Persian Gulf War (PGW) veterans and potential risk factors for adverse health experiences. With the broad question of what adverse health consequences veterans have suffered as a result of their service, the range of relevant experiences is also very broad. The strength of evidence for or against increased risks of specific health outcomes among those who served in the Persian Gulf (PG) depends in part on what research studies have been conducted, and hence on numerous explicit and implicit decisions made by large numbers of research investigators and funding agencies, often acting individually with little perspective on overall needs and priorities. As a result, the research record is of uneven depth and quality. Our task is to summarize the data available to date that appear relevant to our charge of examining possible health consequences of PGW service and to recommend the nature of future studies that would provide more—and better—answers to this question.

Although medical scientists often can use clinical data and individual reports of health experiences to identify areas of concern, such data and reports cannot in themselves provide proof of cause and effect about the health outcomes of PGW service. No matter how well documented an illness may be, or how moving a personal story, unexplained illnesses also occur in the civilian population and in troops not deployed to the Gulf. A basic question regarding the connection between illness in veterans and their service is not whether specific illnesses or adverse health experiences occurred, but whether the frequency or severity of such outcomes was increased over what occurs in otherwise similar populations that were not in the PG.

Battle injuries are universally recognized as a hazard of war. Diseases and infections historically have produced casualties in past wars. Veterans from every war have suffered stress-related symptoms variously known as shell shock; battle fatigue; combat exhaustion; traumatic neurosis; and, since 1980, posttraumatic stress disorder (PTSD). In addition, service members on active duty are subject to the same health hazards as the civilian population, although not necessarily to the same degree: accidents, cancer, heart attacks, stroke, and the like. With the exception of imbedded depleted uranium (DU) fragments and possibly leishmaniasis, very few illnesses or injuries were clearly connected to PG service.

However, this committee was convened, in part, in response to congressional concern that there might be something unique to the PG region or to the war fought there that resulted in specific illnesses, some even becoming manifest long after veterans had left that region. Over time, the military services, the Department of Veterans Affairs (DVA), and other federal agencies have expanded the scope and scientific rigor of investigations into the health of PGW veterans in an effort to systematically develop a body of knowledge about their health experiences and risks associated with exposures described in the previous chapter. The committee and other investigators are seeking to determine whether the risk of illnesses was increased among PGW veterans and what research should be carried out to make such determinations.

In this overview, we make some general observations about the strengths and limitations of the evidence as a whole. The range of possible PGW-related health effects that can be studied at this time is intrinsically limited. Illnesses and symptoms that occurred during the deployment and were transient in nature were not studied or monitored systematically then and are very difficult or impossible to study retrospectively now. For example, possible temporary decrements in lung function associated with exposure to pollutants from the oil well fires were not evaluated at the critical time and are not very amenable to study now, although they may be important.

Likewise, health effects that first come to attention years after the precipitating exposure cannot easily be studied. Many of the known causes of chronic diseases, such as cancer and coronary artery disease, operate over longer periods than have passed since the PGW and, therefore, cannot yet be evaluated in Gulf War veterans. For example, it is commonly believed that most cancers have a minimum 10-year latent period between exposure and detection of the first extra cases of disease. Thus, although no excess adverse cancer effects have yet been reported, delayed effects that have not yet come to light are still possible. What can be examined now are effects that appear early and are persistent or become manifest at some time up to several years after the relevant exposure.

Concerns about unusual illnesses among PGW veterans arose initially through reports of individuals and then through "outbreak" studies, in which teams of epidemiologists studied groups of soldiers who reported a high prevalence of a cluster of symptoms later proposed to be characteristic of a "Gulf War Syndrome."

To provide some support to those veterans concerned about their health, to enable them to receive a clinical work-up, and to gather information on a possible connection to service in the PG, the DVA and the Department of Defense (DoD) created registries and voluntary referral programs for troops, including DVA's National Referral Center and PG Health Registry (PGHR) and DoD's Comprehensive Clinical Evaluation Program (CCEP).

Veterans who have voluntarily participated in these registries have not been found to have any unusual rates of diagnosable conditions (DoD, 1996; Kang, 1996; Kang et al., 1995) but do report a pattern of symptom complaints similar to that seen in the outbreak studies. The registries also share the scientific limitations of the outbreak studies, in that participants are self-selected, symptoms are self-reported, exposures are self-reported and could not be validated, and there is no suitable control group.

Because of these limitations, the committee has concluded that the information on veterans' health that exists in the registries cannot serve alone as a basis for scientific study of the health effects of the PGW. The committee does consider these registries and their affiliated clinical referral programs as useful in assisting veterans who need clinical services and possibly useful as a source of hypotheses regarding the nature and extent of health problems experienced by PGW veterans.

The DVA and various units of the DoD also have undertaken a variety of scientific studies of the health status of PGW veterans. The number and scope of these studies have increased rapidly over the past several years, but few studies had been completed as of May 1996. Findings of several of the completed studies are summarized in this overview. A more complete discussion of these studies and of studies planned or under way is provided in subsequent sections of this chapter, and a listing of research completed, under way, and planned is included in Appendix F. Most of these studies are limited by the absence of detailed exposure information related to individual troops or units. Consequently, studies have had to be designed to seek effects that are sufficiently widespread to be evident when comparing troops who served in the Gulf with those who did not (PG-era veterans).

If an environmental exposure or experience was sufficiently widespread among PGW troops and if the health effects of that exposure were sufficiently severe, effects on mortality rates during and after deployment might be demonstrated. To investigate this question, DoD and DVA individually undertook a study of mortality rates of deployed troops and appropriate comparison groups. These studies of mortality rates during deployment documented the rate of battle-related mortality, and both studies found increased rates of death due to accidents and unintentional injury. Despite isolated findings of slightly increased or decreased cause-specific mortality among the cohort of troops deployed to the PG, the overall finding from these studies was that no disease-specific mortality rate was increased among PGW troops.

In summary, these mortality studies provide no evidence for an increase in total mortality in the cohort of 697,000 PG veterans that is consistent with a common health complaint or exposure, although mortality from accidents and unintentional injuries appears to be increased in the PG veteran group. The information provided is, however, of limited value in identifying the nature and extent of health effects of PGW service. These studies provide no information, of course, on health problems that did not result in increased mortality. Moreover, because the entire cohort of troops or veterans is studied without identification of exposure-based subgroups, these studies are intrinsically insensitive to increased mortality in a subset of troops subjected to a specific, so far unidentified, exposure. Finally, the period of follow-up has, thus far, been only 2 years. If they occurred, health effects of PGW service might not affect mortality rates for many years.

To gather information about morbidity rates among PGW veterans, the Naval Health Research Center (NHRC) at San Diego has undertaken two studies of hospitalization rates, one in PGW veterans who remained on active duty and a second in residents of California who separated from military service after the PGW. Preliminary findings from the first study found no consistent evidence of increased risk of hospitalization for any cause among PGW veterans compared with nondeployed veterans, even after adjusting for a possible healthy worker effect, as suggested by a 10% lower hospitalization rate of PGW veterans prior to deployment.

Strengths of this study included the large sample size, ability to adjust for differences in demographic characteristics of PGW and PGW-era veterans, and completeness of the hospitalization data. Yet this study is also of limited value in assessing the health consequences of the PGW. First, it was not feasible to include any but those who remain on active duty. Evaluation of this limitation may be possible with completion of the study of separated troops residing in California. Furthermore, this second study will permit examination of effects that were not evident until after the PGW. As with the mortality studies, an analysis of hospitalization rates in the entire cohort would be unlikely to detect health effects of exposures that affected a small geographic or occupational subset of the cohort. Nevertheless, the mortality and hospitalization studies, when taken together, provide no evidence of an association between any health experience and environmental exposure of sufficient severity to increase the risk of early death or hospitalization for the entire cohort of deployed troops in the 2-year period after deployment.

Recognizing that mortality and hospitalization rates may not be affected by an increase in the symptoms described in the outbreak studies of military units, investigators have initiated several studies designed to assess the prevalence of self-reported symptoms among PGW veterans and appropriate comparison groups. At this time, only one population-based survey of veterans is nearing completion (Kaiser et al., 1995): a survey of all regular Navy Seabees who were on active duty during the PGW deployment and were still on active duty between September 1994 and June 1995. This study found no differences in measures of physical health or symptom rates between troops deployed to the Gulf (N = 527) and those on duty elsewhere (N = 970). However, Seabee veterans who had been deployed to the Gulf did have higher mean levels of psychological symptom scores. Again, a limitation of this study was the absence of any specific information about exposures experienced by individual troops. The NHRC is now conducting a broader study of active, reserve, and separated Navy Seabees who were on active duty during the era of the PGW.

Psychological sequelae are important and somewhat predictable consequences of service in war. We recognize that they can disable otherwise healthy individuals, but psychiatric diagnoses should not be adopted in default of other medical diagnoses. Furthermore, we believe these are war-related illnesses that deserve attention by the military and DVA in terms of both prevention and treatment. Several studies of stress and responses to stress are described below.

Many veterans have expressed concern about the possibility of adverse effects on their conception of children subsequent to the PGW. Four pilot studies of reproductive health experiences of PGW veterans have been completed, and three large population studies are now under way. None of the four pilot studies have detected increased rates of adverse reproductive outcomes in PGW veterans.

Given the preceding overview, the committee has not identified scientific evidence to date demonstrating adverse health consequences specifically of PGW service other than the documented incidents of leishmaniasis, combat-related or injury-related mortality or morbidity, and increased risk of psychiatric sequelae of deployment. At the same time, the committee recognizes that studies provided to us thus far do not comprise a comprehensive scientific investigation of the health consequences of service in the PGW.

In addition to the recommendations for research given in Chapter 2, the committee believes that value to the military services and the country will result from completion of the NHRC reproductive studies, well-designed scientific studies of determinants of vulnerability (and resilience) to stress arising in deployment and combat, investigations of unexplained illnesses and of relatively obscure syndromes (e.g., chronic fatigue syndrome), and research into improved methods to diagnose leishmaniasis. If proposals for such studies are identified through established procedures for peer review, the committee recommends that they be favorably considered for funding.

We have organized the accumulated evidence by study type and endpoint into the following sections: mortality studies, hospitalization studies, diagnosed diseases in PG veterans, studies of self-reported symptoms (outbreaks and surveys), adverse reproductive outcome studies, mental health studies, and women's health studies. The research activities known to the committee as of May 1996 are listed in Appendix F. We turn now to a review of the epidemiologic evidence.

MORTALITY STUDIES

Records of deaths during the period of deployment are available, and the mortality experience of the PGW veteran cohort, both during and after deployment, is reviewed in this chapter. Death records are uniquely informative and available, in that without taking any special measures, the information is likely to be very nearly complete and accurate regarding the person and the time of occurrence. Even during the PGW itself, both battle casualties (Helmkamp, 1994) and nonbattle casualties (Writer et al., 1996) were comprehensively ascertained.

There is a restriction on the types of events that can be suitably monitored through mortality data. Only fatal injuries can be evaluated, and they may or may not follow the same pattern as nonfatal injuries. Diseases with a high case-fatality rate such as lung cancer can also be evaluated through mortality data. However, for some diseases, death is an unusual consequence; examples are arthritis, asthma, and nonmelanoma skin cancer. Relative to mental health, severe depression may be reflected to some extent in suicide mortality, but mortality data may tell us very little about severe nonfatal psychiatric disorders. Although multiple causes of death are often recorded and coded, the interpretation of nonunderlying causes of death is still difficult and uncertain. Not all potentially relevant ancillary causes will be noted, and the extent of completeness may well vary in relation to social and demographic factors and in relation to the source and quality of health care, including military versus nonmilitary providers.

The adequacy, accuracy, and detail of mortality data are suitable for some assessments of health risk but not for others. In general, broad categories of fatal disease can be examined with some confidence (e.g., coronary heart disease or suicide), whereas death certificate classifications are less reliable for diseases that are more difficult to diagnose or require more specific classification (e.g., the chronic neurologic diseases or subtypes of leukemia).

Two mortality studies of PG veterans have been conducted (Kang and Bullman, 1995; Writer et al., 1996). Both studies encompass general PG veteran populations. Each study includes very large samples. One assessed mortality for veterans up to 2 years after active duty; the other assessed mortality during active duty. Both studies compared troops deployed to the PG with troops deployed elsewhere during the same period. Neither includes information about specific environmental exposures. No excess mortality was observed among PG personnel, with the exception of combat-related deaths and deaths due to accidents and unintentional injury.

We do not consider battle deaths (evaluated by Helmkamp, 1994), although we do evaluate wartime nonbattle deaths (described by Writer et al., 1996). Writer et al. (1996) studied troops with active duty status during or shortly after the PGW. All men and women who were on active duty in the PG theater of operations between August 1, 1990, and July 31, 1991, were identified, with demographic information, dates of service in the PG and elsewhere, and date and cause of death. The control group was composed of service personnel stationed elsewhere at the same time. Among the 1,622 total nonbattle deaths during this year, 1,397 occurred in nondeployed service personnel (73 per 100,000 person-years) and 225 occurred in those deployed (85 per 100,000 person-years). More than half ($N = 967$) of all deaths were due to unintentional injury, with more than half of these ($N = 501$) being motor vehicle injuries. Other major contributors were deaths from illness ($N = 294$), suicide ($N = 216$), and homicide ($N = 103$).

By using the experience of nondeployed veterans to generate expected mortality rates for those deployed, relative risk (RR) estimates were generated, with adjustment for age. The RR = 1.12 (95% confidence interval [CI] = 0.97–1.26) for all nonbattle deaths. This means that there were 12% more deaths in PG veterans than in veterans who had not been in the Gulf theater, but that random variation in the number of deaths is readily compatible with any figure from a 3% decrease to a 26% increase. Since this range includes "no difference," evidence for an effect of Gulf service on total mortality is weak. Similarly, RR = 1.18 (95% CI = 1.01–1.34) for all injuries; RR = 1.54 (95% CI = 1.32–1.77) for unintentional injury; RR = 0.34 (95% CI = 0.16–0.63) for suicide; and RR = 1.15 (95% CI = 0.73–1.73) for a combination of cardiovascular disease and unexpected or undefined causes of death. Subject to the inherent limitations in mortality data noted above and the restricted study period, these data suggest that an increase in unintentional injury was associated with deployment, but most other comparisons were consistent with "no difference."

A second major report concerns mortality in the 2 years after the end of hostilities. PGW veterans were compared with veterans from the same era who did not serve in the Gulf (Kang and Bullman, 1995). This historical cohort mortality study was conducted among all 695,516 men and women who served in the PG between August 1990 and April 1991 and a sample of 746,291 veterans from the same period who served elsewhere, matched by branch of service and unit type (active, reserve, and guard). The interval of follow-up was May 1, 1991, through September 30, 1993, or date of death, whichever occurred first. The investigators identified 1,765 deaths among PGW veterans and 1,729 deaths in the control group. Age was included in the multivariate analysis to control for possible differences in the distribution of this variable between the two groups.

The risk of death was slightly higher among PG veterans who remained on active duty than among other active duty veterans from the same era, with a mortality rate ratio (relative risk) of 1.15. Several causes of death were reduced, but not significantly, among PG veterans, including infectious disease, cancer, and respiratory disease, whereas a consistent pattern of significantly elevated risk was found for unintentional injuries, including motor vehicle injuries, for which the relative risk estimates were around 1.5. Suicide and homicide rates were similar in the two groups.

The overall mortality (RR = 1.47) for female veterans of the PGW was slightly higher than the overall death rate for other women veterans. Investigators also found a significant twofold increase in unintentional injury and motor vehicle injuries, but no significant differences in mortality due to specific illnesses. The relative risks of homicide and suicide were elevated (RR = 2.0 and 1.5, respectively), but these were not statistically significant. The same overall pattern was present but less pronounced among reserves.

Kang and Bullman (1995) compared mortality in both PG veterans and PG-era veterans with that in the total U.S. population of the same age and sex and found that for men, total mortality was markedly reduced among both groups of veterans compared with the U.S. population, as were deaths from unintentional injuries and motor vehicle injuries. Both groups of women veterans showed reduced mortality rates compared to those of the general population, with somewhat elevated rates of suicide and motor vehicle injuries for PGW veterans.

Both of these studies (Kang and Bullman, 1995; Writer et al., 1996), particularly that of Kang and Bullman (1995), point to injury, both intentional and unintentional, during and after the war as the leading cause of excess mortality among PGW veterans. This is not to say that a potential effect on mortality due to illness has been disproved, only that such an effect could not be demonstrated with 2 years of follow-up. This is an important finding, and further follow-up will be appropriate for evaluating possible differences between groups for medical conditions with longer latency periods.

HOSPITALIZATION STUDIES

Computerized hospital discharge data provide a resource for assessing whether PGW veterans were at increased risk of hospitalization after the war relative to appropriate comparison groups and for investigating the distribution of primary diagnoses as defined at hospital discharge. Because hospital discharge data are collected and reported by individual hospitals, which serve poorly defined populations, studies of hospital discharge rates often focus on geographically defined populations, such as persons who report that their permanent residence is in a specified state. Virtually all hospitalizations of active duty personnel take place in military hospitals, and all military hospitals participate in a hospital discharge record system maintained by DoD. However, hospitalizations that occur after discharge can take place in private; public; VA (Veterans Administration); and for those who are retired, military hospitals, making total case ascertainment extremely difficult.

Since the population who served in the Gulf is fairly well defined and a very high percentage of hospitalizations during military service can be recovered among those who remain on active duty, studies of hospital discharge data can provide sound comparisons of hospitalization experience based on large numbers of observations. This minimizes the effect of sampling variability on the findings. Hospitalization records typically provide detailed demographic data that can be used to control for important potential sources of confounding. The data reflect the diagnosis assigned at hospital discharge and are only as accurate as the diagnostic categories used in hospitalization records and the diagnostic evaluations conducted at the hospitals under study. Comparisons of large samples will not provide information about the risk of hospitalization among subsets of the PGW veteran population subject to specific exposures or hazards unless exposed populations can be defined. Additionally, military treatment centers may not provide the majority of care for certain health conditions of interest (e.g., obstetric care is often provided in the civilian sector for some of these military groups). Finally, hospitalization studies of those who remain on active duty will be subject to biased ascertainment if health-status-specific discharge rates differ for PG and PG-era veterans.

To date, one study of the hospitalization experience of PGW veterans has reported preliminary findings (Coate et al., 1995). These investigators, at the NHRC in San Diego, used a retrospective cohort design to compare prewar and postwar hospitalization rates of 547,076 regular Army, Navy, Marine, and Air Force active duty troops deployed to the PG between August 8, 1990, and July 31, 1991, with those of 618,335 nondeployed veterans. The study sample consisted of all regular service personnel on active duty at the beginning of the study period who were deployed during that period and for whom records were available, and a random sample of nondeployed personnel matched for service. Four periods were selected for study: October 1, 1988, to July 31, 1990 (prewar); August 1, 1991, to December 31, 1991; all of 1992; and January 1, 1993, to September 30, 1993. The period August 1, 1990, to July 31, 1991 (roughly the period of the PGW), was not included because of known differences in care between the two groups during that time. In each period, the study was restricted to people who were still on active duty on the first day of the study period. Hospitalization data were drawn from the DoD hospital discharge records provided by all U.S. military hospitals and were matched to records of service personnel by social security number. Hospitalizations for any cause and with a diagnosis in each of 14 broad ICD-9 (International Classification of Diseases, version 9) diagnostic categories were compared for deployed and nondeployed personnel, both before and after adjustment for demographic characteristics.

This study found no increased risk of hospitalization for any cause among PGW veterans compared with nondeployed veterans, even after adjusting for a possible "healthy worker effect." (This is a phenomenon commonly observed in studies of workers, whereby their death and disease rates are lower than those of the general population. Reasons may include favorable health status associated with the ability to find or keep a job, the comprehensive health care offered by some employers, errors in reporting work status, and other factors. In the present context, perhaps it could be called the "healthy veteran effect.") Examination of 14 broad diagnostic categories in each of the three postwar periods found only four instances of possible increased risk of hospitalization among PGW veterans: neoplasms (largely benign), 1991; diseases of the genitourinary system, 1991; diseases of blood and blood-forming organs (mostly anemias), 1992; and psychiatric disorders, 1992. No diagnostic category of hospitalizations was elevated in all three postwar periods. PGW veterans did experience higher rates of hospitalizations for psychiatric disorders. Detailed analysis of these hospitalizations showed an increased risk of hospitalization related to the use of alcohol and drugs.

This study (Coate et al., 1995) had several important strengths. The large sample size and availability of demographic data reduced the effects of sampling variation and confounding on the results. Virtually all hospitalizations of active duty personnel (with the possible exception of childbirth) take place in military hospitals and are captured in the hospital discharge data set, so that bias in ascertainment of hospitalizations is not likely to explain the observed results.

Limitations of the study include its restriction to regular active duty personnel who remained on active duty throughout the study period. Of the initial cohort of 1,279,931 individuals, 91% remained on active duty on August 1, 1991; 84% remained on January 1, 1992; and 66% remained on January 1, 1993. Increased hospitalization rates among those who left active duty because of their illnesses would not have been detected unless these illnesses had led to hospitalization prior to discharge. Diseases with latency periods longer than 3 years would not be detected by this study, nor would illnesses that did not lead to hospitalization. Increased hospitalizations due to public awareness of the putative Gulf War Syndrome would have been limited to PGW veterans. Since this was not observed, response bias appears not to have appreciably affected the data.

The team at NHRC also is conducting a study of rates of hospitalization of veterans from all service branches who have separated from active service. This study will compare the hospitalization rates of PGW veterans and a random sample of PGW-era veterans in nonmilitary hospitals in California between 1989 and 1994. The PGW cohort will be defined as military personnel who deployed to participate in the PGW at any time between August 2, 1990, and July 31, 1991. The study population will be further limited to PG veterans who, when deployed, had resided in California for at least 1 year. Prewar hospitalization rates will be collected to compare the predeployment health status of PGW and PGW-era veterans. Hospitalization rates also will be compared to those of active duty personnel.

This study has the potential to complement the previously described hospitalization study of the same group of PGW veterans who remained on active duty. It will address the possibility that PGW veterans experiencing adverse health effects of service were differentially separated from service, thereby masking a health impact on the cohort as a whole. The study will provide information on hospitalization rates after separation for about 12% of the PGW cohort, the percentage of troops who satisfy the California residency requirements. Limitations of the study include its inability to identify hospitalizations outside California for the same individual and the possibility that admission criteria differ for nonmilitary hospitals and VA Medical Centers (VAMCs). Despite these limitations, this study will provide information about hospitalization rates after discharge that complement the previously described study of PGW veterans who remained on active duty after the war. It may also help to characterize the potential for differential follow-up in the study of military hospitalizations resulting from earlier separation of veterans experiencing health problems after the war. This is a good plan that may provide a model for future deployments.

It will be important for researchers to acknowledge study design limitations as they interpret the findings. A limitation of both mortality analyses and hospital discharge analyses as commonly performed is that they are usually restricted to a single cause of death on the certificate (usually the "underlying cause of death") or a "principal reason for hospitalization." A second limitation of both study designs is that even an examination of the entire PGW veteran cohort would be unlikely to detect the health effects of exposures that affected only a small geographical or occupational subset of the cohort or were rare events. When taken together, however, completed studies of mortality and hospitalization rates of PGW veterans provide no evidence of an association for any widespread or common environmental exposure or other threat to health of sufficient severity to increase the risk of early death or hospitalization among a large segment of the cohort of deployed troops in the 2 to 3 years after deployment.

DIAGNOSED DISEASES IN PG VETERANS

One disease that has been diagnosed in a small number of veterans is leishmaniasis. As discussed in Chapter 2, the diagnosis of viscerotropic leishmaniasis is difficult to make, and only 12 cases of the viscerotropic and 19 cases of the cutaneous form have been diagnosed among PG veterans (Hyams et al., 1995). Leishmaniasis has been associated with service in the PG.

DoD and DVA have established registries to which active duty service personnel (DoD) and veterans of the PG war (DVA) can report any illnesses or symptoms that they believe are related to PGW service and receive a health review and examination according to a standard protocol. Associated with each of the registries are follow-up centers that provide more extensive examinations as needed. Since 1992, DVA has had three national referral centers—in Washington, D.C.; Houston, Texas; and West Los Angeles, California. In 1995, a fourth referral center was added at the VAMC in Birmingham, Alabama. The DoD Specialized Care Centers (SCCs) offer, in addition, medical treatment and rehabilitation services. Both registries were established to provide veterans with health concerns access to comprehensive physical examinations and baseline laboratory and other appropriate diagnostic tests. These registries could be used to identify individuals with illnesses and symptoms that may have resulted from service in the PG. However, because both registries were designed to provide a clinical series of self-referred persons for whom common health-related information is collected systematically, they are not suitable for use in formal studies of the frequency of PGW-related adverse health effects.

Both registries and their related referral centers continue to operate and to register additional self-referred individuals. Besides providing service to individuals who attend the health review and follow-up exams, these registries provide minimal ongoing morbidity surveillance.

Public Law (PL) 102-585 included instructions to the secretary of Veterans Affairs to establish and maintain a PGHR, whose purposes and nature were not specified in the law. As indicated in the committee's first report (IOM, 1995a), the PGHR may be a valuable clinical tool, but it was not designed to provide information on etiology or disease frequency and cannot be used alone for research on these matters. As also indicated in the committee's first report, registry data are computerized, but considerable lag times remain from data collection to data entry to availability of data for review and use. The data collection instrument was modified and fully fielded in 1996 to allow reporting of up to ten complaints and diagnoses, where three had previously been the maximum. If there is an error or omission in completion of the form, it is rejected at the point of data entry and returned to the field for correction. Although this quality control check is important, the rejection rate is high and contributes to the slow turnaround time. As a consequence, recently collected data are not fully compatible with data collected earlier, particularly when reporting "any illness." Data reviewed and reported to the committee through January 1996 still contain no more than three symptoms or diagnoses. We review these data below, but caution that base rates and comparisons are subject to considerable potential bias.

DVA Persian Gulf Health Registry

Data from the DVA PGHR have been analyzed separately for women (*N* = 5,429) and men (*N* = 46,784). Nine of the ten most frequently reported complaints were the same for men and women (Table 4-1). Of those with symptoms, a diagnosis was made for 77% of women and 77% of men. Men and women without a diagnosis after examination reported fatigue, headache, skin rash, muscle and joint pain, memory loss, shortness of breath, sleep disturbances, chest pain, and diarrhea (Table 4-2). Women reported abdominal pain among the 10 most frequent symptoms, whereas men reported cough.

As seen in Table 4-3, men with a diagnosis more frequently had infectious diseases and circulatory system diagnoses, whereas women more frequently had genitourinary system diagnoses. Whether these genitourinary diagnoses among women are related to the relative unavailability of gynecological care in the Gulf theater cannot be determined, but may warrant further consideration. Regardless of symptom or diagnosis status, 69% of women reported their health as all right, good, or very good compared with 73% of men (Kang et al., 1995).

Table 4-1. Ten Most Frequent Complaints of Female (*N* = 4,919) and Male (*N* = 42,705) Veterans in the Persian Gulf Health Registry with Complaint Data Available

Complaints(s)	Women (%)	Men (%)
Fatigue	23.3	20.7
Headache	23.0	17.7
Skin rash	18.2	18.5
Muscle, joint pain	14.5	16.5
Loss of memory and other general symptoms	13.9	14.2
Shortness of breath	7.6	8.0
Sleep disturbances	5.3	5.9
Abdominal pain	3.9	2.5
Other symptoms involving skin and integument	3.8	3.2
Diarrhea and other gastrointestinal symptoms	3.6	4.5

SOURCE: Data were received May 1996 from the DVA Environmental Epidemiology Service for registrants through January 1996 (Kang, 1996).

Table 4-2. Ten Most Frequent Complaints of Female (*N* = 1,009) and Male *N* = 8,705) Veterans in the Persian Gulf Health Registry with Symptoms but No Diagnosis

Complaint(s)	Women (%)	Men (%)
Fatigue	31.5	29.5
Headache	30.3	21.4
Skin rash	20.8	19.8
Muscle, joint pain	15.4	15.6
Memory loss	14.5	15.5
Shortness of breath	10.1	9.6
Sleep disturbances	5.8	6.6
Chest pain	3.9	4.9
Diarrhea and other gastrointestinal symptoms	3.4	3.8
Abdominal pain	3.3	3.0
Cough	3.2	4.3

SOURCE: Data were received May 1996 from the DVA Environmental Epidemiology Service for registrants through January 1996 (Kang, 1996).

Table 4-3. Distribution of Diagnoses for Female (*N* = 4,919) and Male (*N* = 42,725) Veterans in the Persian Gulf Health Registry

	Women		Men	
Diagnosis	No.	%	No.	%
Musculoskeletal/ connective tissue	1,128	22.9	10,763	25.2
Mental disorders	839	17.1	6,198	14.5
Respiratory system	825	16.8	5,974	14.0
Skin/subcutaneous tissue	619	12.6	5,719	13.4
Nervous system	474	9.6	3,438	8.0
Digestive system	464	9.4	4,938	11.6
Genitourinary system	440	8.9	1,134	2.7
Infectious diseases	224	4.6	3,144	7.4
Injury and poisoning	212	4.3	2,016	4.7
Circulatory system	203	4.1	3,109	7.3
Neoplasm	18	0.4	179	0.4

SOURCE: Data were received May 1996 from the DVA Environmental Epidemiology Service for registrants through January 1996 (Kang, 1996).

DoD Comprehensive Clinical Evaluation Program

In June 1994, DoD developed a clinical protocol, based on the one being used by the DVA, to provide a comprehensive health exam. Active duty service members who were PGW veterans were encouraged to refer themselves. In 1995, DoD established a Specialized Care Center at Walter Reed Army Medical Center to provide intensive treatment to symptomatic veterans. Referrals for this intensive 4-week treatment are accepted from clinicians who identify individuals that are unable to perform their duty or meet fitness and retention standards.

In August 1995, DoD published the results of the first 10,020 participants in the CCEP (DoD, 1995). That report and the June 1995 draft were analyzed extensively by the Institute of Medicine (IOM) Committee on the DoD Persian Gulf Syndrome Comprehensive Clinical Evaluation Program. This committee, separate from ours, was established in July 1994, at the request of DoD. Its evaluation noted that the principal shortcoming of CCEP exams was that they were "not, however, designed to answer epidemiological questions. Instead, it was designed as a medical evaluation and treatment program" (IOM, 1996, p. 2); however, the committee recognized the "compassionate and comprehensive effort to address the clinical needs of thousands of active duty personnel" (p. 1). Finally, the committee made several recommendations designed to improve the quality of the clinical information obtained.

The most recent evaluation of CCEP data summarizes the completed diagnostic results of 18,598 participants (DoD, 1996), addressing concerns indicated in the IOM (1996) report. CCEP participants include a greater percentage of women, blacks, and older persons than their actual representation in the total deployed PGW force.

The data from this report are subject to limitations, as DoD clearly has recognized and reported. The CCEP was designed as a clinical rather than a research program; the findings are subject to selection bias since persons had to agree to be evaluated, symptoms are self-reported, reported exposures cannot be validated, and there is no comparable control group. The findings are summarized in Tables 4-4 and 4-5.

One significant advance in military medicine was generated by this program, according to the CCEP report (DoD, 1996). DoD has implemented a comprehensive medical surveillance program for U.S. forces in Bosnia, incorporating lessons learned from the CCEP. The information gathered prior to deployment will allow for better assessment of any subsequent health problems. Stress management programs will be made available to service members and their families. These efforts may help to prevent or reduce the development of illness, psychosocial problems, and other adverse conditions that could result from deployment of U.S. service members in future combat and military operations.

Table 4-4. Twelve Most Cited Complaints and Their Frequency as Chief Complaint Among 18,075 CCEP Participants

Complaint	Reported as "Any Complaint" (%)	Reported as "Chief Complaint" (%)
Joint pain	49	11
Fatigue	47	10
Headache	39	7
Loss of memory	34	4
Sleep disturbance	32	2
Rash/dermatitis	31	7
Difficulty concentrating	27	<1
Depression	23	1
Muscle pain	21	1
Diarrhea	18	2
Shortness of breath	18	3
Abdominal pain or gastrointestinal symptoms	17	3

SOURCE: DoD, 1996.

Table 4-5. Frequency of Primary Diagnosis Among 2,131 Female and 15,944 Male CCEP Participants and Frequency of Any Diagnosis for All 18,075 Participants

Primary Diagnosis	Women (%)	Men (%)	All Participants, Any Diagnosis (%)
Psychological conditions	19.1	18.3	36.0
Symptoms, signs, and ill-defined conditions	16.5	18.1	43.1
Musculoskeletal system diseases	15.9	18.6	47.2
Nervous system diseases	8.8	5.3	17.8
Healthy	8.6	9.9	10.2
Respiratory system diseases	6.1	6.9	17.5
Skin and subcutaneous tissue diseases	6.0	6.3	19.9
Digestive system diseases	4.9	6.5	20.4
Genitourinary system diseases	3.6	1.0	5.4
Endocrine diseases	2.7	1.9	7.9
Infectious diseases	2.5	2.6	9.0
Circulatory system diseases	1.6	2.3	8.0

SOURCE: DoD, 1996.

The DoD is currently in the process of making the CCEP database available for use by outside investigators, with all identifying information on individuals in the database removed. The details of accessing these data were not available at the time this report was being finalized, but may be available from DoD by the time this report is released.

Predictors of Enrollment in the Persian Gulf Health Registry

The availability of databases containing information on Army soldiers, including Army reserve and National Guard, who were deployed to the PGW theater and the information on those who registered in the DVA PGHR have led to an investigation of possible determinants of registration. A population of 50,000–60,000 Army soldiers (including reserve and National Guard) who deployed to the PG in Operation Desert Shield/Storm will be identified, including registrants in the PGHR and three controls for each registrant who deployed to the Gulf but who, at the time of analysis, had not registered. All personal identifiers are to be removed, and results presented in aggregate. This study uses information available from DVA and DoD to describe, very roughly, the kinds of individuals who are entered on the PGHR. Variables to be examined among these groups for a possible association with registry enrollment include demographic, medical, and health risk behaviors. The investigators indicate two main objectives to this exercise: (1) to evaluate the techniques and statistical methods necessary for combining and analyzing medical and demographic records before, during, and after deployment; and (2) to determine differences between soldiers enrolling and not enrolling in the registry. Hypotheses for future studies will be generated and information can be used to identify soldiers at risk for reporting problems. This could allow for development of possible interventions before deployment, thus reducing risk. It will be important for the analyses to group factors into exogenous (age, gender, race, and distance from nearest VAMC) and endogenous (disease) categories and to study relative influences. If data are available on whether a registrant or control has health coverage, and its type, information may be generated on the importance of this variable for registry participation. We encourage a substantial increase in statistician involvement in this study.

STUDIES OF SELF-REPORTED SYMPTOMS

Outbreak Studies

Studies in which investigators focused on reported clusters of symptoms or illnesses among PGW veterans are similar in many respects to the frequent "cluster studies" of illness in the U.S. with a possible environmental cause

(Caldwell, 1990). This analogy is instructive because many of the investigators who have participated in such cluster studies have become skeptical about their scientific value (Rothman, 1990) (also called outbreak studies or "hot pursuit" studies, characterized as fast, preliminary investigations). The typical cluster study is characterized by small sample size, selection problems (i.e., many other groups could have been studied but were not, because the participants did not report a cluster), poorly identified exposures, and a significant potential for information bias resulting from respondent awareness of the underlying concern.

In the environmental domain, these studies rarely have been fruitful (Bender et al., 1990; Cutler et al., 1986). A few well-done cluster studies can be useful at the early stages of an investigation to help define the problem and to rule out some statistical flukes that have been misinterpreted and some possible etiologies. That phase of research on the reported Gulf War Syndrome has been completed. Exploratory studies failed to generate useful leads about either the condition or the exposures that might cause such a condition.

This report reviews three such studies: the 123rd Army Reserve Command (DeFraites et al., 1992), the Reserve Naval Mobile Construction Battalion 24 (Berg, 1994), and a unit of the Pennsylvania National Guard (MMWR, 1995; Reeves, 1995). In each case, the unit came to medical attention because of a report of what appeared to be an unusually high rate of unexplained illness. The troops were then carefully studied by a medical and epidemiologic team.

123rd Army Reserve Command (ARCOM)

The first "hot-pursuit" study was completed by investigators at Walter Reed Army Institute of Research (WRAIR) (DeFraites et al., 1992), who investigated reports of symptomatic complaints among reservists belonging to the 123rd ARCOM, Lafayette, Indiana. Staff of the 123rd ARCOM Surgeon's Office became aware of these complaints early in 1992. Similar complaints were reported subsequently by members of the 417th Quartermaster Company, in Scottsburg, Indiana.

In response to growing concern about these reports, the team from WRAIR visited Fort Benjamin Harrison and neighboring facilities in April 1992. During this visit, 79 reservists who were concerned about their health were evaluated. All 79 participants completed a medical questionnaire, and 78 completed a Brief Symptom Inventory (BSI) and were available for a detailed interview. Each reservist interviewed completed a brief psychiatric intake-type interview and had vital signs measured. All but one of the reservists received a dental examination. All 78 who participated in the interviews also had blood drawn for complete blood count, white blood cell differential, platelet count, erythrocyte sedimentation rate, and liver function studies. All sera were tested for antibodies to *Leishmania tropica*. The performance characteristics of this test for use in screening have not been fully defined (DeFraites et al., 1992). Sera from selected individuals were tested for antibodies for brucellosis. Limited comparative data were available from other groups of veterans.

Fatigue was the most common symptom (70%). Other systemic symptoms, including fever, abdominal pain, and diarrhea, were less common. The onset of fatigue and associated symptoms tended to occur after redeployment from the PG; the onset of diarrhea was more frequent during deployment. No cases of leishmaniasis, brucellosis, or Lyme disease were detected. The findings did not suggest a common pattern of illness among study group members.

Review of potential exposures during Operation Desert Shield/Storm (ODS/S) provided no evidence that the respondents had exposures to microwaves, chemicals, radiation, or other suspected environmental hazards. These reservists did report high levels of stress. Investigators noted that the rapid deployment and subsequent redeployment were stressful for many reservists and their families. They believed, however, that PTSD was present in few, if any, of these reservists.

The investigators concluded that this study provided no objective evidence of an outbreak of any diagnosable disease in this group. They concluded that the documentable medical problems and illnesses found were typical of a general population with similar demographic characteristics. As investigators noted, this study provided no basis for defining a "case" of disease. No evidence of a common exposure was found.

DeFraites et al. (1992) reported that symptoms and objective findings seemed to appear in two peaks, one coincident with return from the Gulf and another some 6–8 months later. They could find no calendar month associations, clustering by activities, or evidence of any "dose-response" relationships with increasing length of time in the Gulf theater to suggest that at least some of the reported symptoms could be related to the reentry of these reservists. The largest proportion of illnesses that resulted in time lost from work was attributed to injuries and, thus, was recognized and explained. The morbidity assessments reported in this investigation do not include data collected by civilian providers, so only a portion of the health records are available for a limited subset of participants.

This study is useful in documenting the absence of a common underlying malady or environmental exposure among a group of reservists who initially appeared to have similar medical problems. It also shows that the complaints of this group did not represent a common pattern of illness or environmental exposure. Somewhat reassuring, however, was the fact that one of the first studies of aspects of a PGW-related illness did not show alarming patterns of disease or exposure, other than the possible impact of stress on the troops.

Reserve Naval Mobile Construction Battalion 24 (Seabees)

The second investigation reported by DoD involved the Reserve Naval Mobile Construction Battalion 24 (Seabees) (Berg, 1994). Many members of detachments of this battalion complained of symptoms that they believed were related to their service in the Gulf theater. The Asheville, North Carolina, detachment first reporting symptoms was contacted in November 1992, and additional detachments of this Seabees battalion were followed a year later.

A team of physician epidemiologists and a preventive medicine technician visited four detachments of the unit between November 1993 and February 1994 to evaluate Seabees who believed they were affected by PGW-induced health problems. A total of 154 of 232 ODS/S veterans in four detachments were surveyed. After investigators obtained proper consent from the reservists, diagnoses were verified by medical record review and by interviews of medical care providers.

The findings centered on the evaluations of these 154 ODS/S reservists. These veterans reported from 1 to 20 symptoms, including fatigue, joint and muscle pains, and confusion and irritability, but the symptoms did not point to a common underlying medical diagnosis. This study did not identify patterns of disease or exposure that seemed to be useful to define further research.

Pennsylvania Air National Guard

In December 1994, the Centers for Disease Control and Prevention (CDC) began an investigation of a report of unexplained illnesses among veterans of the PGW who belonged to a unit of the Pennsylvania Air National Guard. The initial cluster investigation expanded into a study being conducted in three stages. The first stage focused on the identification and characterization of the signs and symptoms of disease in these troops. The second stage was designed to compare the frequency of symptoms in PGW veterans and guardsmen who had not been deployed to the Gulf. The third stage was designed to characterize the illness and identify risk factors. A further discussion of each stage follows.

Stage 1. A team of CDC medical epidemiologists visited the VAMC and surveyed primary care physicians and regional hospitals in south-central Pennsylvania, identifying 59 veterans reported to be symptomatic. These veterans were evaluated by standardized interviews and physical examinations. They were found to have a high prevalence of symptoms considered to be moderate or severe, including fatigue (61%), joint pain (51%), nasal congestion (51%), diarrhea (44%), joint stiffness (44%), unrefreshing sleep (42%), and a variety of others suggestive of mood disturbances and musculoskeletal disorders. No consistent abnormalities were identified on physical examination (MMWR, 1995).

Stage 2. From January to March 1995, 3,927 members of the index unit and three comparison units were surveyed. This survey established that in all units, symptom rates were higher in veterans who had been deployed to the Gulf than in those not deployed. Symptom prevalence was greater in the index unit than in the comparison units; however, the index unit had nearly twice the deployment rate of the comparison units. Controlling for deployment accounted for the apparently higher rates in the index unit (MMWR, 1995; Reeves, 1995).

The investigation then focused on identifying case-defining symptoms. Two approaches were used: clinical epidemiologic and statistical. In the epidemiologic approach, a symptom was considered case defining if it had been present for 5 or more months, was reported by at least 25% of PGW veterans, and was reported at least 2.5 times more often by PGW veterans than by those not deployed. This approach yielded three clusters of symptoms: (1) fatigue; (2) mood and cognition disorders (impaired memory or concentration, moodiness, or difficulty sleeping); and (3) musculoskeletal complaints (joint stiffness or pain). The statistical approach employed factor analysis to identify two symptom factors. The first was characterized by fatigue and impairment of mood or cognition; the second was characterized by joint or muscle pain and joint stiffness. The epidemiologic and statistical approaches produced similar findings, and investigators focused on the epidemiologic approach. Based on these findings, they proposed a working case definition of illness as one or more chronic symptoms from two or more of three symptom categories: (1) fatigue, (2) mood and cognition, and (3) musculoskeletal. Preliminary findings by CDC investigators found that 42% of PGW veterans and 13% of nondeployed troops in the study met the working case definition. Investigators concluded that this symptom complex was very common among PGW veterans, whereas the prevalence rates were similar for nondeployed veterans and a civilian population involved in a study of chronic fatigue syndrome (Reeves, 1995).

Stage 3. This stage will compare cases, using the working case definition above, and controls from the Air National Guard unit to identify possible risk factors. The proposed study design includes provisions for structured questionnaire administration, structured physical examination and specimen collection, and proposed medical record review. Stage 3 was not complete at the writing of this report.

Investigators concluded from the observations to date that the statistical and epidemiologic approaches yield highly concordant working case definitions for a definable syndrome, which can be used to define severity of illness based on the severity of underlying symptoms. They also concluded that the syndrome defined in this way is common in PGW veterans but is also found in nondeployed members of the Air National Guard.

Summary

These studies came to the similar conclusion that troops reported high rates of a variety of nonspecific symptoms, including fatigue, joint pain and stiffness, disturbed or unrefreshing sleep, some gastrointestinal complaints, and a variety of complaints suggestive of mood and musculoskeletal disorders.

Although these studies demonstrated considerable similarity in the nature of the reported health problems across units, they had limited ability to determine the existence or nature of a unique Gulf War Syndrome. First, because these studies were initiated in response to reports of unusual medical problems in the three units, they do not provide information about the prevalence of such problems in the larger cohort of troops deployed to the Gulf.

Because symptoms are self-reported, it is difficult to determine whether the higher rates represent true differences or whether they result from recall bias among troops aware of the general public debate about a Gulf War Syndrome as well as the medical concerns of others in their unit. There is also the possibility of an increased rate of reporting among troops sensitized to notice and bring to medical attention minor and transient symptoms, in part because of concern about the availability of health coverage and eligibility for DVA medical care on a "service-connected" basis should those symptoms become more severe.

A second concern is that the outbreak studies have not consistently linked these symptoms to either a medical diagnosis or a specific exposure. Investigators were severely limited in their ability to associate symptoms with exposures in the Gulf since military records were not designed to maintain this type of information and no common exposure was evident among those interviewed.

A third concern is that the symptoms reported in these units are also common in the general population (Kroenke and Price, 1993). When a study population is selected because of a reported cluster of affected troops and no scientifically valid comparison group is available, the investigation cannot provide a scientific basis for determining whether rates of self-reported symptoms differ from those expected in the general population of military veterans, or in the population at large, by more than random variation. Certain factors are also known to influence symptom perception fairly dramatically, including cognition (beliefs), context (setting in which the person has a symptom), attention (degree paid to it), and mood (Barsky, 1995).

Thus, although these outbreak studies were successful in demonstrating a common pattern of perceived health problems across a range of military units deployed to the Gulf, they were not successful in demonstrating that these symptoms occurred at a higher rate among PGW veterans than among PGW-era veterans, or that these symptoms could be linked to specific medical diagnoses or exposures. Proposals for future studies of this type should be scrutinized carefully; they are unlikely to be useful, and they may divert attention and resources away from potentially more useful studies.

Surveys

This section reviews the results of several surveys of PGW veterans and comparison groups. In some studies, the survey was supplemented by examination of all or a subset of study participants. These studies provide information on the frequency of self-reported symptoms and illnesses of soldiers deployed to the Gulf theater and may be of value in identifying diagnoses or illnesses of special concern. The major limitation of such studies is that they reflect the respondents' reports of perceptions of their health status, and such reports commonly reflect more than health per se. To the extent that responses are influenced by reporting and public discussion of the health effects of the PGW, individual reports may not correspond to the findings that would be obtained by medical examination. Even if the possibility of reporting bias is taken into account, however, well-designed surveys can provide information about the number and characteristics of veterans who, by their own assessment, do have specific illnesses or symptoms.

There are good reasons to achieve consistency in format and style, but those reasons do not necessarily define the most scientific approach to studies that depend on symptom lists and questionnaires or that use subjective psychological interviews. The most important reasons for consistency are to better ensure the utility of results and the robustness of findings for cross-collaboration with other studies. However, judgments about exactly how to achieve such consistency must remain with the scientists designing the studies. From time to time, under the mandate of the Reduction in Paperwork Act and its general charge to protect both the public and the public purse, the Office of Management and Budget (OMB) has required consistency in the questions included in a wide variety of survey instruments. However, changes in the thrust of the research projects have resulted sometimes. Substantial delay in initiation of some potentially important research has occurred. OMB should give high priority to rigorous and timely PG research by ensuring that DVA, DoD, and other agencies make adequate and appropriate use of scientific review by expert peers and encourage the development of individual study designs.

Naval Health Research Center (NHRC) Studies

At this time, initial findings from only one population-based survey of veterans of the PGW have been reported (Kaiser et al., 1995). This was a survey of all regular Navy Seabees who served in the Gulf or elsewhere at the same time and were still on active duty between September 1994 and June 1995. A total of 1,497 Seabees responded to the survey, 527 of whom had been deployed to the Gulf. The Seabees were selected for study because Mobile Construction Battalion 24 had previously reported a high prevalence of symptoms, and the more current work built on these initial investigations (Berg, 1994).

The demographic characteristics of deployed and nondeployed respondents were similar. Veterans who had been deployed to the Gulf had higher mean scores on all five dimension scales of the Hopkins psychological symptoms profile (somatization, obsessive-compulsive disorder, interpersonal sensitivity, anxiety, or depression); higher scores indicate greater severity or extent of symptoms. Their mean scores were low relative to the mean scores of patients with clinically diagnosed depression or anxiety disorders. Active duty Seabees are concentrated in California and Mississippi, and investigators traveled to those sites during the study period. The reliability of the study instrument was evaluated through retesting 260 study participants on a subsequent visit. For a random sample of 150 of the 260 participants in the reliability study, medical and service records were obtained and compared to survey responses. Physical measurements of grip strength and spirometry were obtained for study participants. Mean values of grip strength and FEV1/FVC ratio (ratio of forced expiratory volume in one second to forced vital capacity), a measure of airway flow, did not differ between Seabees who went to the Gulf and those who did not.

An outside panel reviewing the studies at NHRC was skeptical that a study of active duty Seabees was adequate to address PG health issues, due to the number of Seabees that did not remain on active duty because they were in the reserves or separated from service. Therefore, a more comprehensive study has been designed to investigate self-reported post-PGW symptoms of physical and functional illness among all Navy Seabees (active, reserve, or separated from the military) who were deployed to the PG between August 1, 1990, and June 3, 1991. The symptom rates will be compared to those of PG-era veterans. The population identified for this study includes all men and women Seabees (approximately 17,500) who served at least 1 month during the interval specified.

For this cohort, baseline information and a determination of physiological and psychological events and syndromes will be assessed by a telephone interview and follow-up database searches of hospitalizations and mortality. Initial analyses will examine participation rates, questionnaire data (descriptive), and questionnaire data in conjunction with the geographical information system (GIS). Investigators plan to track study participants using the Defense Manpower Data Center (DMDC) database and will obtain death certificates from the DVA or National Death Index (NDI).

If an acceptable response rate is obtained from the initial survey, the study will proceed to Phase II surveys, with periodic reanalysis of follow-up data in the years 2001, 2006, and 2011. Because the population is relatively young and healthy, investigators do not anticipate sufficient numbers for hypothesis testing until the later study years.

This is a reasonable study, although it is disappointing that the study was not initiated by DoD several years ago. The main drawbacks are problems with the telephone survey, overstudying of the Seabee population, incomplete follow-up, and data capture in general. Refusal bias is another major threat. The investigators have indicated that they will document correlates of refusal; in this way, they will know whether the study is valid, but there is no reliable way to protect against these sorts of biases.

Although the study is restricted to Seabees, they constitute a well-defined target population; it has the potential to be informative, but exposures will be self-reported. Findings and associations detected in specific study populations may serve to define needs for studies of other PG veteran populations.

DVA National Health Survey

The National Health Survey of PG veterans and their family members, funded by DVA, is a mailed survey that will compare self-reported prevalence of health outcomes between 15,000 PG and 15,000 PG-era veterans randomly selected from the DMDC database, oversampling for women and reserve troops. Exposure data will be self-reported and, eventually, linked with DoD unit location files. At the time of this writing, surveys have been mailed and a repeat mailing has been sent. This study may have adequate power for certain relative risks to eliminate associations if participation rates are high and if recall bias can be ruled out. The investigators, in their proposal, comment on many of the issues and threats to validity.

This a well-designed and well-intended study, but it has started at least several years too late. Recall problems and the inability to obtain accurate information on those who died before the study started are major threats to its validity. If the response rate is low, if there is a strong differential in the propensity to participate between PG veterans and PG-era veterans, or if there is differential recall bias, the study will be limited. There appeared to be little statistical input in the analysis plan reviewed, and these data will require sophisticated statistical adjustment. The survey instrument is well formatted to increase completeness and accuracy. However, symptom checklists can be of questionable value. Definitions are fuzzy, and higher prevalences can arise when checklists are used than when respondents are invited to report their symptoms without a checklist.

Additional aspects of the DVA study include a validation study, special efforts to reach a sample of nonrespondents, and physical examination of both PG and PG-era veterans. The review of military records is a good idea, but if the record and the questionnaire disagree, which is the gold standard? Inviting these individuals for physical examination is a major undertaking and may or may not provide useful information on health outcomes. Investigators should address what they will do if in fact the validation study shows that study results may not be valid.

Survey of Iowa Veterans

A smaller survey of PG veterans (approximately 3,000) is being conducted in Iowa, funded by CDC at the request of Congress. Study objectives are to determine differences in the prevalence of health outcomes between (1) PG veterans and PG-era service personnel; (2) PG active duty military and non-PG active duty military; (3) PG National Guard and reserve troops and non-PG National Guard and reserve troops; and (4) PG active duty and PG National Guard and reserve troops. The protocol is a comprehensive document. The level of detail indicates what is intended and how tasks will be accomplished. The project will have three advisory committees: internal, external scientific, and external community.

The statistical power analysis indicates that the study can detect a 50% rate increase in the "exposed" group; exposure is not specified but is assumed to be "service in the PG." Available information on health consequences indicates that a 50% increase may be unrealistically high. The actual power of the Iowa study to detect a smaller increase will be substantially lower than the 80% indicated in the analysis. The survey methods proposed include a 5% reinterview rate that will allow estimation of interview reliability.

Despite this study's strengths, it has two major limitations. First, the telephone interview is critical to the entire approach. There are problems inherent in trying to collect the necessary information by telephone self-report. In addition, the interview will be long; there will be many who refuse to participate, and others will terminate the interview part way through. Because of these factors, the sample will be highly selected. Information collected from surrogates is likely to be very different from that obtained directly from study participants.

A second and greater concern is that this study has been limited to Iowa. Much work has already gone into a study that will be underpowered and too narrow. Sample size calculations were based on examining "risk" among those exposed versus those not exposed (presumably exposed or not exposed to the PGW). Because it is likely that subpopulations or less than the whole study group will be of interest for analyzing outcomes, the study is unlikely to have adequate size to detect significant differences. The population of Iowa veterans is also likely to be too narrow a focus because veterans with an Iowa home of record may differ in some explained or unexplained way from the total population of PG veterans, which will limit the interpretation of results. The "Iowa" constraint is very limiting.

ADVERSE REPRODUCTIVE OUTCOME STUDIES

Pathways for Environmental Influences on Reproduction

The following section on reproductive outcomes and methods for studying them is purposely more detailed than other sections in this chapter, to serve as an example of the methodologic difficulties involved in a specific area of research, which can be broadly applied to other study designs. Its length is not meant to reflect or imply a greater degree of importance of this potential health outcome.

To study reproductive health consequences of PG service and determine the potential for further productive research, one must consider how environmental exposure might exert such effects. These pathways or mechanisms help to define how reproductive health might be influenced by some aspect of having served in the PGW.

One possible mechanism for adverse effects on reproduction is through direct harm to the nonpregnant woman, such as genetic damage to the ovum, which can lead to chromosomal anomaly in the fetus (Kline et al., 1989), or scarring of the fallopian tubes, which leads to an inability to conceive (Healy et al., 1994). These changes, although permanent, may not be detected for many years after they have occurred, until the woman attempts conception, pregnancy, or delivery. Other types of direct harm may be temporary or reversible.

Males also may have adverse reproductive effects from exposure to environmental agents. Exposures that damage sperm production can produce temporary or permanent infertility (Schrader and Kesner, 1993; Skakkebaek et al., 1994), and some types of genetic damage to the sperm could result in fetuses or children who do not develop normally (Olshan and Faustman, 1993). Since the production of sperm cells is continuous throughout adult life, most genetic damage that affects spermatozoa directly will be manifest only in pregnancies conceived relatively soon after the exposure (within about 74 days) (Scialli, 1992). Thus, male exposures related to the PGW that were soon followed by conception would be most plausibly affected in this manner. It is possible for stem cells to be permanently harmed, although they appear to be less susceptible than later stages of spermatogenesis (Scialli, 1992). If they do undergo genetic changes, however, these would result in continuous production of genetically defective sperm. Exposures that produce this effect would lead to a permanent decrease in fertility or an increase in risk of abnormalities in the offspring.

Most research on the reproductive consequences of environmental exposures in general has focused on pregnant women and, hence, on exposure of the fetus. There is abundant evidence that the fetus is highly vulnerable to insults that come through the pregnant woman (Shepard et al., 1993), with potential increases in a range of different adverse outcomes. If severe harm early in pregnancy causes miscarriages prior to the recognition of pregnancy, the woman is likely to be misdiagnosed as infertile. Fetal loss at a later stage results in miscarriage or stillbirth. These are generally recognized and reported, although definitions of miscarriage versus stillbirth versus postpartum death are difficult to apply consistently. Thus, differences in reported data may simply reflect differences in reporting standards.

Structural damage to the developing fetus can result in congenital malformations, whereas reduced growth and low birth weight may reflect a range of fetal insults. Preterm delivery can be a consequence of either maternal or fetal problems. A lengthy interval between maternal exposure and fetal effects can occur only if the maternal exposure itself is persistent, which may occur with exposure to heavy metals or chlorinated hydrocarbons that persist in the bone or fat of the mother and cause a sustained elevation in blood levels. The relatively small number of pregnancies among women while they were serving in the Gulf limits opportunities to study immediate fetal effects, but the potential for continuing effects of a persistent maternal body burden of Gulf-related toxic agents needs study.

Definition of Outcomes

Many facets of reproductive function have been associated with exposure to drugs, chemicals, and other environmental agents (Mattison, 1994), ranging from loss of libido to failure of spermatogenesis or lactation to major birth defects. Many of these reproductive events are difficult to define and diagnose accurately. Infertility is, in part, a function of the opportunity to conceive and, thus, is likely to remain undetected for some time, perhaps long after biological damage has occurred. Miscarriages are notoriously difficult to identify with certainty, readily missed when they occur early in gestation, and potentially overdiagnosed when menstrual periods are unusually heavy or delayed (Kline et al., 1989). Many congenital anomalies cannot be detected at birth or in very young infants, and accurate and complete diagnosis requires careful examination at the proper time in development. Congenital heart defects, for example, are rarely identifiable in live newborns and require monitoring the child for up to 5 years to be comprehensively ascertained.

Because there are often no standardized definitions and the number of identified reproductive events depends on the level of scrutiny, valid research designs must identify the frequency of adverse outcomes in truly comparable groups with and without exposures. For example, given the lack of standardization in the definition of miscarriage, there is no benchmark or "normal" rate of miscarriage to which an exposed population may be compared. Instead, an exposed population must be compared with an unexposed population, with the same miscarriage definitions and the same opportunities for observation of miscarriage. Conditions subject to underascertainment require comparable levels of scrutiny in the populations to be compared: infertility rates will appear higher in a population that has a greater desire to have children than in a population that has less desire simply because failures to conceive will come to attention more often in the former.

As another example, about 5% of all newborns can be found at the time of birth to have abnormalities, increasing to about 10% after the first year or two as problems become manifest, but many of these may be diagnosed only by a specialist experienced in this field. Findings in an exposed population subject to special searching are not comparable to findings in an unexposed, unscrutinized population. Even the term "congenital defect" encompasses a wide range of processes, including DNA damage of parental germ cells prior to pregnancy, adverse intrauterine environment, and birth injury. Much of the scientific literature on environmental exposures and reproductive outcomes has been based on studies of special, often high-risk, populations. Thus, direct comparisons of rates of adverse outcomes in those special studies with the rates among PGW veterans may be misleading.

Some male veterans and their partners have reported that contact with their semen causes a burning sensation in the partner. This issue was discussed at some length by an expert panel convened by the Department of Veterans Affairs (DVA, 1995a), with efforts to identify how many such cases had been reported, whether any known condition could account for such a phenomenon, and what might be done to further evaluate the reports. Based on a few case reports of allergic responses to seminal constituents (Bernstein et al., 1993), the most plausible candidate explanation for this symptom is some type of local hypersensitivity reaction. This hypothesis is based on the absence of male discomfort associated with seminal fluid and the temporal pattern of symptoms after exposure to ejaculate.

Dr. David Bernstein, an immunologist at the University of Cincinnati Medical Sciences Center, reported to the panel that detailed evaluations of approximately 40 couples as described in the scientific literature are consistent with this phenomenon. The women complain of allergic symptoms after exposure to semen that are not accounted for by infection, which is a much more common explanation for such symptoms. Symptoms are prevented by use of condoms, and in some cases the hypersensitivity has been treated successfully.

In theory, such a phenomenon could be induced by male exposure to agents that contribute to the formation of new allergens in the seminal fluid. However, as noted by the panel, there is no clear documentation at this time of how frequently the phenomenon is reported by either veterans or the general population. The recommendation of the DVA's expert panel for a clear case definition followed by accurate information on the magnitude of the problem among PG veterans is a reasonable approach.

Frequency of Events in the General Population

Many of the broad categories of reproductive problems are quite common, with typical ranges for infertility of 10% of all couples, and 10–15% of recognized pregnancies resulting in fetal loss (perhaps 30% or more including those not recognized), and with 5–10% of those resulting in preterm delivery or low birth weight. Even congenital malformations, which are individually rare (less than 1 per 1,000), are not as rare in the aggregate, being recognized in 3–5% of infants at the time of birth. Congenital malformations range from cosmetic (birthmarks or webbed toes) to significant impairment (Down's syndrome or congenital dislocation of the hip) to severely life threatening or lethal (aneuploidy, anencephaly, or transposition of the great vessels). Thus, anecdotal case reports of a given exposure (whether associated with the PGW or with a drug or environmental chemical) must be interpreted very cautiously because of the high baseline rate of adverse reproductive outcomes.

For many reproductive outcomes, not all individuals in a given population will contribute information. In a population of exposed and unexposed individuals, only a subset will attempt to conceive (needed to address infertility), a subset of those will have conceptions (needed to address miscarriage rates), and a subset of those will result in births (needed to address birth weight or congenital malformations).

Reports of clusters of adverse reproductive outcomes (particularly miscarriages or birth defects) have often come to attention as possible clues to a hazardous environmental exposure. None of these episodes of reported clusters in the general population have yielded new insights into the causes of reproductive health problems, in spite of many investigations by health departments, CDC, and others. Often, despite what appears to be an unusual number of events, the small population of interest—with the resulting limited opportunity to examine dose-response gradients and confounding—leaves these episodes unresolved. In addition, once potentially affected individuals become aware of and concerned with that possibility, they are often more attentive to potential hazardous exposures and adverse outcomes and may be inclined to report more exposure and more disease (perhaps more accurately) than comparison populations, so that further reports of an excess must be questioned. Therefore, especially in light of heightened awareness, nothing short of a rigorous evaluation of exposures, reproductive outcomes, and potential confounders is likely to yield informative results.

Confounding

Much like the healthy worker effect, in which mortality rates are reduced in employed populations due to screening and selection of physically and mentally fit individuals, there may well be a healthy soldier effect that applies to reproductive outcomes. Screening to participate in the armed services and further selection to serve in the PGW may have produced a population with above-average reproductive health as well as good general physical health and, hence, with a lower-than-normal expected frequency of reproductive health problems. For example, persons with some kinds of hereditary defects may be excluded from military service. Studies intended to address potential adverse effects of exposures in the Gulf theater must take such selection into account, perhaps by identifying equally fit military populations that did not serve in the PG.

Another phenomenon that has been observed in groups of employed women is the selection of populations that have not had live births (i.e., continued employment of women who have been infertile or had pregnancy losses) since those who had live births tended to leave employment (Lemasters and Pinney, 1989; Savitz et al., 1990). Thus, those who remained in the work force more often had an unfavorable reproductive history as a result of factors unrelated to their work. An analogous phenomenon might occur in studying women in the military: those who fail to conceive or conceive but fail to deliver a live birth may be most likely to remain on active duty, even if the reproductive problem had origins before or unrelated to military service.

A number of "life-style" exposures are known to influence reproductive health, including the use of tobacco, alcohol, and illicit drugs; diet; and sexual behavior involving the risk of sexually transmitted infections. Studies must take such risk factors into account in trying to isolate any effect of the PG experience per se. Service in the Gulf may have affected these behaviors during and after the war, so that isolating the effects of environmental agents encountered during the war on reproductive health requires measurement and adjustment for behavioral risk factors.

Given such considerations, national surveys such as the National Health and Nutrition Examination Survey or the National Maternal and Infant Health Survey may not provide suitable standards to evaluate rates of outcomes for comparison to PGW veterans.

Reproductive Outcome Studies in PG Populations

Pilot Studies

Although many studies of PGW veterans are in progress, four pilot projects have evaluated the possibility of adverse reproductive health experiences, and three larger population-based studies are under way. The pilot projects include studies of: (1) birth defects among children born to veterans from four Mississippi National Guard Units (Penman et al., 1996); (2) pregnancy outcomes among veterans at Robins Air Force Base (Eggert, 1994); (3) miscarriage rates in the William Beaumont Army Medical Center population (Rosa, 1993); and

(4) analysis of miscarriage rates at six Army hospitals (Broadnax, 1992), comparing the proportions of pregnancies ending in miscarriage prior to and after the war. Each of these studies found no pattern of adverse reproductive effects from which hypotheses could be generated.

In sum, inferences about the effect of some aspect of service on reproductive health are not warranted at this time. Perhaps the strongest conclusion that can be drawn at present is that no ubiquitous exposure associated with PGW service has been found to produce an adverse impact on common reproductive outcomes.

NHRC Studies

A study of the reproductive health of veterans is currently in progress at the NHRC in San Diego. A multifaceted study of the health of PGW veterans ("Epidemiologic Studies of Morbidity Among Gulf War Veterans: A Search for Etiologic Agents and Risk Factors") includes three projects focused on reproductive outcomes: (1) "A Comparative Study of Pregnancy Outcomes Among Gulf War Veterans (Male and Female) and Other Active Duty Personnel"; (2) "Reproductive Outcomes"; and (3) "Prevalence of Congenital Anomalies Among Children Born to Gulf War Veterans."

The first project, comparing birth defects among offspring born in military hospitals to deployed versus nondeployed veterans, has been presented in preliminary form (Cowan et al., 1995). Active duty personnel who were deployed to the PG (approximately 580,000) and a sample of troops not so deployed (approximately 700,000) were identified and followed to identify live births in military hospitals. The study included all births conceived after return from the Gulf by deployed persons and after January 1, 1991, by nondeployed persons. Date of birth was on or before September 30, 1992. Outcomes examined were live birth rates, birth defects, and infant sex ratio.

Nearly 16,000 live births occurred among spouses of deployed men and 18,000 among spouses of nondeployed men; approximately 2,000 live births occurred to deployed women and 5,000 to nondeployed women. Birth rates were similar for men who were and were not deployed (29.1 versus 29.6 per 1,000), as well as for deployed and nondeployed women (56.4 versus 59.5 per 1,000). Sex ratios (male to female) were in the range of 0.99–1.06 for all groups, well within the expected range for samples of these sizes. Discharge diagnosis codes for offspring of active duty veterans who had been deployed in the Gulf showed birth defects in the range of 7% for offspring of men and 9% for offspring of women. Relative risks comparing deployed to nondeployed men and women were 1.02 (95% CI = 0.94–1.11) and 1.13 (95% CI = 0.97–1.32), respectively, prior to adjustment for known differences in confounders. These relative risks did not depend in any systematic way on duration of service in the PGW. Adjustment for race, age of mother, branch of service, and rank reduced relative risk estimates for both men and women (RR = 0.98 and 1.04, respectively).

Preliminary results of this study provide no evidence for any major association between simple deployment in the Gulf and birth defects in the aggregate. They do not address specific exposures encountered in the war or specific birth defect outcomes, nor do they address the experience of veterans who are no longer on active duty or who had a child born outside of a military hospital.

The second NHRC study focuses on self-reported infertility and miscarriage based on a mailed survey to be sent to married couples. The sample includes strata in which women served in the Gulf, men served in the Gulf, women served in the military but not in the Gulf, and men served in the military but not in the Gulf, with 4,000 to be chosen from each of the four groups. All couples will have been married at least 1 year, and the sample will include active duty, reserve, and nonactive duty personnel. The survey includes demographic factors, life-style, medical history, contraception, reproductive history, and other environmental exposures. Study plans include repeated mailings of the questionnaire, with telephone follow-up to improve response rates.

Based on a review of the questionnaire and study plans, the methods seem to be carefully developed and suitable for addressing the endpoints of infertility and miscarriage, despite the considerable challenges in eliciting accurate data on miscarriage and other outcomes. The instrument is brief and designed to encourage complete and accurate reporting. Plans for follow-up of nonrespondents are likely to be successful. The overall design is well suited to screen for potential adverse effects on fertility and pregnancy outcome.

The third study of reproductive health focuses on congenital abnormalities in the offspring of veterans. Although this outcome was considered in the hospitalization study, the third study will include more complete information from birth defects registries for evaluation of any association with PGW experience. Records of veterans who served in the PGW and those who did not will be linked to population-based registries of birth defects in Arizona, Arkansas, Hawaii, Iowa, Oklahoma, Georgia (Atlanta), and California (selected counties), each of which has an active monitoring program in place. Births to veterans who lived in these states will be identified from birth certificates, which will allow linkage to the birth defects registry. In addition, there are plans to examine fetal deaths, birth weight, and gestational age using vital records. The proportion of births with specific adverse outcomes, such as malformations or low birth weight, will be compared among PGW and PGW-era veterans, as well as with the nonveteran populations in those states. Approximately 9,500 live births are expected to have occurred to PGW veterans in the selected states.

This is an ambitious study for this research team, proposing to conduct record linkage on a scale not previously attempted in the United States. Investigators are conducting a large-scale feasibility study in Hawaii to evaluate study methods. If feasible, the strategy is a good one for studying the overall birth prevalence of malformations. Even though there may be incomplete identification of all births to PG veterans ("all births" serving as the denominator for the calculation of adverse outcomes), the actual proportion of infants with adverse outcomes may not be affected. Within the groups of births identified as having occurred among PGW and PGW-era veterans, the birth defects registries should be quite effective in comprehensively ascertaining and diagnosing early malformations. Despite the study's limitations, the proposed study, if feasible, will be a reasonable approach to a broad survey of congenital defects in the offspring of PGW veterans.

Based on a review of the protocols, critique by a panel of independent experts, and response from the team of investigators, some general characterization of the set of projects can be made. Subject to practical constraints (budgets and feasibility), quality of data sources (medical records and self-report), and selection of subsets of all possible reproductive outcomes for detailed study, the projects represent a reasonable set of choices. Through this series of studies, investigators will be able to consider infertility, miscarriage, low birth weight, preterm delivery, and congenital malformations.

It is critical to note, however, that unless there are major modifications, investigators will address a potentially broad or universal effect of PGW service rather than specific exposures. Although the global hypothesis of some PGW effect is less precise than one or more specific hypotheses about exposure to individual agents, no highly specific hypotheses are now considered to have much scientific support, and a global view is a reasonable starting point. If results are positive, they could be used to identify more refined issues for further study.

Overall, the ongoing efforts to address reproductive health appear to be responsive to the broad and somewhat diffuse array of present concerns. Without some particular, focused hypothesis for a specific environmental agent or outcome, there seems to be little need for expansion beyond the present effort. If the results of those studies provide specific leads to an increased risk of particular outcomes, such leads should be pursued with more detailed research and larger samples to evaluate exposures encountered in the war. It is also possible that some specific exposures producing known reproductive health consequences will be identified as having occurred, which would warrant more focused study of reproductive outcomes. However, unless a broad effect or some specific exposures associated with adverse reproductive effects are identified, there is little reason to continue research on the reproductive health consequences of service in the PGW beyond what is now planned.

MENTAL HEALTH STUDIES

The mental state of troops is an important dimension of military effectiveness because it both reflects and affects unit cohesion, morale, and leadership. DoD has invested in programmatic research, focusing on the stressors associated with deployment, as well as the mental and physical well-being of PGW-era personnel. The DVA also has conducted several studies of the health of veterans beginning with their return home (NEPEC, 1992) and continues such research through activities based at specific VAMCs.

Issues in Studies of Mental Health

Investigators have begun to study some of the questions concerning the mental health of PGW veterans and possible associations with service in the PG. To do so, they have had to address several issues challenging all researchers studying mental health. Measurements of mental health phenomena rely strongly on subjective perceptions of events, emotional responses to them (how one feels about a life experience), and cognitions (how one thinks or gives meaning to an experience). For research purposes, the subjective dimensions of an individual's experiences must be assumed to be valid for that individual. Objective indicators of mental health that can be observed by another person are included in mental health assessments: for example, behavior, such as the ability to function in one's work and social interactions; demeanor; test performance; and the like. To promote valid and reliable mental health diagnoses, the American Psychiatric Association (APA) has defined research and diagnostic criteria for psychiatric diagnoses that represent consensus among many experts in the field and has published them in its *Diagnostic and Statistical Manual of Mental Disorders* (DSM) (APA, 1987, 1994). As the field of mental health has developed, diagnostic criteria and the nosology of diagnoses have been continually refined. One such example is PTSD, a phenomenon that has been described in conjunction with prior wars but was not named PTSD in the DSM until 1980. Most studies of PGW soldiers produced psychiatric findings that were based on criteria for diagnoses such as PTSD.

It has been noted that one of the difficulties in analyzing mental health scores for tests and scales used in the research described is that the "norms" to which comparisons are made have not been developed for a population of men or women in the military. The nature of many of the scales may have the tendency to show high scores (more illness) for military populations compared with the general population because of the way some questions are phrased (Marlowe, 1996).

Diagnosis of psychiatric problems upon return from the Gulf may capture many of the mental health problems that originated during ODS/S or were exacerbated by service. It could be assumed that troops deployed in ODS/S were mentally fit for duty at the time. However, unless baseline predeployment data are available, it is difficult to discern which problems were present before deployment and did not change significantly, which originated with or were exacerbated by service, and which were worse after return. To complicate diagnosis, some problems are acute and remit quickly; some are chronic; still others have a delayed presentation, that is, they may not be apparent until months or years after return from the theater.

Mental Health Problems and Military Experience

PTSD has become a mental health outcome of primary interest since the Vietnam War era. Many veterans who served in Vietnam were exposed to shocking or horrifying events associated with the war and, in its aftermath, returned to a hostile environment in the United States. Cumulative experiences with "combat stress" after service during earlier wars and growing recognition of the multiple presentations of illness (acute, chronic, or delayed) and sequelae led to recognition of a syndrome (often called "traumatic neurosis") associated with severe trauma. In 1980, the American Psychiatric Association first formulated PTSD among its diagnoses of anxiety disorders in DSM-III. A revision, published in 1987, known as DSM-III-R, was the version used for the studies reported herein (APA, 1987). The version in current use is known as DSM-IV and was published in 1994 (APA, 1994).

Four criteria are listed for PTSD diagnosis in DSM III-R: (1) exposure to an event that would be stressful to almost anyone; (2) one or more specified symptoms of reliving the traumatic experiences (nightmares, intrusive thoughts, or flashbacks); (3) three or more specified symptoms of withdrawal, avoidance, or numbing of emotions; and (4) two or more symptoms of hyperarousal, such as exaggerated startle or difficulty concentrating. A diagnosis of PTSD requires that criteria 2 through 4 have been met during the previous month.

In addition to PTSD, military personnel are subject to other psychiatric disorders including depression, anxiety, substance abuse, and (rarely) a major mental illness such as schizophrenia. These have been documented in some assessments completed by DVA-sponsored projects. In comparison with the attention given PTSD, little detailed information is available on other mental health problems resulting from service in the PGW.

Mental Health: Comparison of Deployed and Nondeployed Troops

A diagnosis of PTSD is usually made by means of a clinical interview, but algorithms have been developed to identify persons likely to have PTSD by using data obtained by questionnaire, such as the Impact of Event Scale (IES) or the Brief Symptom Inventory (BSI). The latter approach allows an approximation of risk for PTSD in large sample studies where clinical interviews are not feasible. The IES is a 15-item scale used to assess reactions to trauma and related characteristics associated with stress disorders. The IES scale emphasizes two dimensions of PTSD, intrusion and avoidance (Horowitz, 1986). High scores indicate more severe reactions to stressors.

In a comparative survey, conducted in 1993, of PG active duty personnel and reserve troops from Hawaii and Pennsylvania, reserve troops scored higher than active duty troops on the avoidance and intrusion scales of the IES, but their scores were remarkably lower than those of active duty personnel in the XVIIIth Airborne Corps and the VIIth Corps, who were studied in 1991–1992 and who had engaged in main-force actions during the ground war. These lower scores in the Pennsylvania and Hawaii samples may reflect attenuation due to passage of another year since ODS, a difference in combat exposure, or other unidentified factors (USAMRMC, 1994).

The BSI is a 53-item scale of symptoms derived from the 90-item Symptom Check List-90-Revised (SCL-90-R) (Derogatis and Melisaratos, 1983). It includes nine dimensions or subscales: somatization, obsessive-compulsive, interpersonal sensitivity, depression, anxiety, hostility, phobic anxiety, paranoid ideation, and psychoticism, as well as three global indices of pathology, including a General Severity Index (GSI). Higher scores indicate more severe symptoms. Of concern in interpreting the results is that military samples differ somewhat from civilian samples. For example, a "normal" military sample might not appear the same as a "normal" civilian sample of nonpatients for reasons specific to military selection (Stretch et al., 1996).

A comparison of BSI scores for active duty and reserve personnel who were deployed to the Gulf versus those who were not deployed indicated that the former were at greater risk of PTSD as assessed using the GSI of the BSI. In addition, the nondeployed active duty personnel of the XVIII Airborne had relatively high scores (USAMRMC, 1994), perhaps reflecting concerns over the unit disestablishments in Europe and turbulence and downsizing in the continental United States.

A PTSD risk algorithm was developed from the IES and BSI and used to identify those at moderate and high risk for a diagnosis of PTSD. Criteria included exposure to a traumatic event outside the range of normal human experience, intrusive thoughts and memories associated with the trauma, symptoms of persistent avoidance of stimuli associated with the trauma, and persistent symptoms of increased arousal associated with the trauma.

Although the ground war was short, scores indicating moderate or high risk of PTSD were more common among those who were deployed than among the nondeployed. Scores of those deployed in the VIIth and XVIIIth Corps indicated moderate to high risk for PTSD in 13–15% of these troops, respectively (studied 6 months to 1 year after ODS), compared with 8% for active duty troops and 10% for reservists from Pennsylvania and Hawaii (studied 2 years after ODS) (USAMRMC, 1994).

Reservists who served in ODS were compared with those deployed in the continental United States and in Europe. Data collected in 1993 revealed that mean scores on a trauma scale constructed from the BSI and the GSI/BSI were essentially the same for personnel deployed in those two areas but significantly lower than scores for the group deployed to the Gulf theater. Thus, activation by itself did not seem to account for psychological symptom levels, which were connected specifically to deployment to the Gulf (Marlowe, 1995).

Inpatient psychiatric services at a U.S. Army combat support post reported no increase in hospitalizations during 1990–1991 by active duty soldiers, families, and retirees before, during, and after ODS/S, coincident with return from ODS. However, the psychiatric proportion of all hospitalizations increased among soldiers not deployed who had served less than 1 year (Koshes and Rothberg, 1994).

In addition to DoD studies, DVA initiated several studies of veterans shortly after demobilization. A summary of the DVA assessments of 9,090 veterans seen through its readjustment counseling service after ODS/S (from May to September 1991) indicated a prevalence of PTSD of 2.2%, subdiagnostic PTSD of 6.4%,[1] and other psychological problems of 3.1%. Prevalence of alcohol or drug abuse was 1.7%, and marriage and family problems were 3.9% (Blank and Gelsomino, 1992).

Site-specific studies of mental health problems among returning veterans revealed a range of prevalence of PTSD across sites. At the New Orleans VAMC, PG troops assessed within the first year after return from war zone duty had prevalence estimates as high as 16–19% (Sutker et al., 1992). At the Boston VAMC, the prevalence estimate was 4% for men and 9% for women according to the Mississippi Scale (Wolfe et al., 1992c). One would expect differences across geographic areas due to differences in exposure to combat and differences in military occupational specialty, as well as differences in the demographic makeup of the populations studied and their desire for health services or counseling relative to that expressed by troops evaluated at other VAMC sites. Results of first-year findings from various VAMC studies have been compiled (NEPEC, 1992). We emphasize that many of these studies were small, several did not have control groups, and others were of self-selected study samples.

[1]Subdiagnostic PTSD includes veterans who meet some but not all of the DSM-III-R diagnostic criteria for PTSD.

Factors Associated with Mental Health Problems: Combat and Other Stressors

A variety of factors have been associated with mental health problems experienced by troops deployed to ODS/S. Although combat exposure is among these stressors, a variety of other stressors were greater after deployment to the Gulf theater than to other sites. For example, troops experienced prolonged disruption of normal living patterns and relationships, reunion and readaptation, and culture shock upon returning from the Gulf. These factors have been studied among active duty and reserve personnel and are reviewed in Chapter 3 of this report.

Factors Increasing Vulnerability to PTSD and Other Psychiatric Disorders

Although combat exposure has a strong influence on development of PTSD, the majority of troops exposed to combat or other major stressors did not develop PTSD. Thus, assessment of vulnerability may aid understanding of how to prevent or attenuate the likelihood of developing PTSD. Vulnerability to mental health problems has been related to person–situation interactions in the psychology and psychiatry literature. A range of factors has been associated with individual differences in response to some stressors; among these factors are ethnicity, gender, educational level, intellectual sophistication as it affects coping, and military rank.

Both Sutker and Wolfe studied the relationship between vulnerability factors and mental health outcomes. Sutker et al. (1993) found in one study ($N = 215$) that female gender and nonwhite race were associated with modestly greater risk of development of PTSD symptoms. In a larger series ($N = 912$; 653 deployed to the PG and 259 with stateside duty), Sutker et al. (1995a) found that race was not significantly associated with depression. Likewise, Wolfe et al. (1993) found that race was not associated with a higher prevalence of mental health problems. Women had a higher prevalence of PTSD symptoms than men in both the Boston and the New Orleans studies (Sutker et al., 1993; Wolfe et al., 1993). Higher educational level and officer versus enlisted status were associated with a lower prevalence of PTSD (Wolfe et al., 1993).

A variety of explanations have been offered for these associations. Education and intellectual sophistication may enhance the soldier's ability to understand events, to garner necessary support through social interaction, and to come to terms with the events of the war. In addition, officer status is associated with greater access to personal and social resources, including better training with which to deal with traumatic experience. Officers are generally older and often more experienced in war or in training for war than enlisted personnel.

Explanations for gender differences in mental health have included the likelihood that women are socialized to express symptoms whereas men are socialized to suppress expression. Another explanation is that women's experiences of trauma in war were different from those of men. This explanation may be warranted by consideration of data about abuse. As discussed in Chapter 3, an experience unique to women or at least much more prevalent among women who served in the Gulf was exposure to violence and sexual harassment (Wolfe et al. 1992b). Those who reported assault had higher Mississippi Scale scores for PTSD symptomatology, and those reporting assault or physical harassment had higher GSI/BSI scores. There is also evidence that past exposure to violence and abuse, such as childhood sexual or physical abuse, is associated with PTSD.

Marlowe (1995) concluded that one could not determine from data collected by DoD whether there were factors that predisposed one to a highly stressed response to combat. He did note that those who were highly stressed before combat were also highly stressed after combat and that those with high psychological symptom scores at the time of the first postcombat study tended to have high scores a year later. These same individuals had high reactions to current life events as well as to ODS events.

Factors Enhancing Resilience or Buffering Effects of Stress on Mental Health

Sutker et al. (1995b) compared 97 PGW troops with PTSD diagnosis to 484 without psychological distress to determine differences in their personal resources (gender, education, intellectual sophistication, and personality dispositions such as hardiness and coping styles) and environmental resources (perceived social support and family relationship support). She found that less commitment, more avoidance of coping, less family cohesion, and lower social support satisfaction were factors associated with those who developed PTSD diagnoses.

DoD studies indicated that the service person's military unit served as a social support mechanism to buffer the effects of exposure to acute and chronic stress on health. Postcombat sharing of experiences within studied units provided a source of aid for coping with the sequelae of war. Shared coping with traumatic events in the field seemed to be more beneficial to soldiers than dealing with such events after returning to the United States (demobilization) (WRAIR, 1992). As identified by active duty troops deployed to the Gulf from Pennsylvania and Hawaii, sources of support that were somewhat helpful included family, friends, chaplains, and unit members. For reserve troops, similar sources of support were indicated. That report (USAMRMC, 1994) stated that more than 90% of active duty and reserve troops studied were coping moderately to extremely well 2 years after ODS/S, but 7.8% of the active duty deployed felt that they were coping poorly versus 5.5% of active duty nondeployed.

Long-Term Mental Health Outcomes

Most studies to date have been of short-term acute outcomes. DVA-sponsored studies discussed above, conducted by Wolfe at the Boston VAMC (Wolfe et al., 1993) and Sutker at the New Orleans VAMC (Sutker et al., 1993), indicated persistence of psychological distress among troops for at least 1 year after return from ODS/S. Marlowe (1995) of DoD has followed selected troops for as long as 2 years after return from ODS/S and found that those who were highly distressed before combat were also highly distressed after combat. Thus, these studies have made significant contributions, but follow-up so far is too short to resolve questions about factors associated with the persistence of PTSD symptoms and other types of illness. Symptoms of PTSD in some veterans have persisted for at least two decades after the Vietnam war.

Physical Symptoms and Exposure to Stressors

Physical symptoms in conjunction with stressors were also studied by DoD. Although physical symptoms do not in themselves signify PTSD or other mental health problems, there is a large literature linking acute and chronic life stress and mental health to future physical morbidities, including gastrointestinal and hyperimmune diseases (Vogt et al, 1994). A comparison of physical symptoms experienced by deployed and nondeployed active duty and reserve troops indicated that those deployed were more than twice as likely to report head colds, sinus trouble, sore throat, difficulty swallowing, headaches, back problems, stomach upset, muscle aches, aching joints, cough, chills or fever, and other problems. This was the case when demographic factors such as age, rank, education, marital status, and branch of services were controlled (Stretch et al., 1995).

An algorithm of physical and psychological symptoms was calculated as a proxy indicator for Gulf War Syndrome (GWS) symptoms (Stretch et al., 1995). These included headache, stomach or intestinal upset, muscle aches or cramps, aching joints and bones, weight loss or gain, cough, chills or fever, general level of spirits, level of energy, trouble with memory, pains in the chest or heart, low energy, difficulty getting breath, difficulty concentrating, and feeling weak in parts of the body. Those reporting five or more of the health symptoms and at least one of the psychological symptoms were identified as follows: 178 of troops deployed (12%) and 55 (2.2%) of those not deployed scored high on this index. Of those with high scores on the GWS index, 42% attributed their health problems to ODS/S service, 45% had concern over exposure to oil fires, 36% claimed to have been exposed to oil fires, and 30% met the criteria for possible

PTSD diagnosis (Stretch et al., 1995). The authors indicate that the most powerful factor discriminating these multiple-risk groups from those not at high risk was whether or not individuals had been deployed to the Gulf.

Investigations by Wolfe and Sutker also addressed the prevalence of somatic symptoms or symptoms with a bodily referent (i.e., pertaining to the body rather than to emotion) among veterans studied immediately after return to the United States and 1 year later. The associations among physical symptoms, stress, and mental health were examined in ongoing studies of Fort Devens reservists. Wolfe et al. (1994) found that women veterans with PTSD ($N = 40$) reported significantly more health symptoms than their counterparts without PTSD ($N = 153$). The following symptoms were reported by 85–100% of women with PTSD, in decreasing order of prevalence: trouble concentrating, depression, nervousness, lack of energy, aches or pains, insomnia, headaches, loss of interests, and crying easily. Those with PTSD also reported more combat exposure, less current social support, and more postdeployment life stressors. When all health symptoms were included in a regression model, anxiety and PTSD were significant predictors of health symptoms, but combat exposure was not. Of interest is that PTSD symptoms of emotional numbing and physiologic hyperarousal were significantly related to the number of health symptoms reported.

Understanding the connection between psychological and physical symptoms and their relation to exposure to traumatic events requires consideration of the temporal ordering of events and plausible mechanisms. Given the lack of predeployment data for most troops, it is difficult to ascertain the temporal order of events. Some may have experienced traumatic events prior to deployment (e.g., rape or sexual or physical abuse), and some may have had prior illnesses with mental and physical symptoms. The DoD and DVA studies document the cooccurrence of stressors (e.g., combat exposure), PTSD-like symptoms, and physical symptoms, many of which are nonspecific. (Chapter 5 of this report addresses consideration of somatization, chronic fatigue, and multiple chemical sensitivity [MCS]). Those with PTSD after ODS/S have had more severe health symptoms (Stretch et al., 1995; Wolfe et al., 1994).

One of the mechanisms proposed to link traumatic events (stressors) with symptoms is the physiologic changes induced as part of the stress response. Studies dating from Selye's classic experiments (Selye, 1956) link stress to changes in the hypothalamic–pituitary–adrenal (HPA) axis hormones, resulting in an increase of glucocorticoid production from the adrenals. Cortisol and other glucocorticoids initiate suppression of immune, metabolic, and neural defensive reactions in response to stress. Over the past two decades, physiologic alterations in response to extreme stress have been studied in humans with PTSD related to a variety of traumatic events (combat exposure, holocaust survivors, rape victims, and survivors of natural disasters). A series of studies of hormonal alterations in response to stress has demonstrated persistent biological changes after extreme stress. Findings of lower basal cortisol levels in people with PTSD are opposite to those expected as part of the normative stress response and suggest possible exhaustion of the response. In contrast, exposures of PTSD patients to a novel environmental stressor and exacerbation of comorbid conditions are associated with elevated cortisol levels. Similar responses occur to acute treatment interventions that involve "reliving" exposure to the stressor (Yehuda et al., 1993). Other studies of PTSD related to abuse show elevated levels of norepinephrine, epinephrine, dopamine, and cortisol (Lemieux and Coe, 1995). Studies of women who have been sexually assaulted show an increased risk of both medically explained and unexplained symptoms (Golding, 1994).

Studies of civilian populations in the Gulf also demonstrate somatic responses to stressors in the war. A telephone survey of the Israeli civilian population found that 38% had somatic reactions to the orders to wear gas masks and move into sealed rooms, but only 20% had somatic responses 12 days later, suggesting adaptation to stress through time. A complex pattern of relationships between expectations about chemical warfare and somatic interactions was evident. Those with specific expectations about future chemical attacks were more likely to have a somatic reaction. Also, women were more likely to react than men. Habituation occurred quickly (Carmeli et al., 1991). In another telephone survey conducted during the third week of the war, 28% of community residents complained about sleep: 10% had awakenings, 4.5% had difficulty falling asleep, and 13.5% experienced both. Women and persons with less education reported more sleep problems (Lavie et al., 1991).

Although PTSD may have psychophysiological components, to date the committee has found no published studies linking PTSD with physiologic aspects of stress response or symptoms with physical referents among ODS/S veterans. Future studies elucidating the psychophysiological consequences of extreme stress and their relationship to both mental health and symptoms with bodily referents are needed.

Discussion of Mental Health Issues

In addition to the literature reviewed above, the committee discussed several psychosocial variables that could influence the incidence of unexplained illnesses among PGW veterans. These included the role of suggestion in shaping symptoms and the role of concerns regarding health care. Also discussed were various psychiatric syndromes that include physical symptoms, PTSD, and other psychiatric outcomes, with recognition of the facts that psychiatric diagnoses are not to be made by exclusion and that they are often comorbid. Each is discussed briefly here.

Many pervasive and powerful suggestive influences have affected PGW veterans, including attention by the news media, Congress, and peers. Reports in the news media, meetings of veterans groups, and public and congressional hearings have served to draw attention to certain symptoms that may be present in PGW veterans or certain possible exposures. These are strong influences affecting patients' recall and reporting. How such forces affect the symptoms reported is not known, but this could be an important topic to evaluate.

Veterans of the PGW returned to a nation in turmoil over health care and its financing. A key question for many veterans was whether DVA would provide the necessary treatment on a service-connected basis; this fear may have been put aside to some extent when legislation determined that unexplained illnesses were service connected, whereas many diagnosed diseases were not. However, this also meant that having a diagnosis did not guarantee treatment if the illness was not considered service connected, especially for reserve and National Guard troops who were left to prove the connection.

Some persons suggested to the committee that certain known syndromes and physical illnesses could explain some veterans' undiagnosed illnesses. How these syndromes and illnesses may or may not be connected to purely physical versus psychiatric diagnoses is not well determined in either the scientific literature or the medical community. Some of these hypotheses are discussed later in this report.

PTSD may be the most studied and expected of the war-related psychiatric illnesses, but there are others that could be manifest in less well defined ways. Our society has a greater acceptance now than in years past of stress as a cause of impairment, as well as a greater tendency to provide compensation for such impairment (e.g., disability claims, legal settlements, and medical retirements). After the Vietnam War, veterans were more forthcoming than previously in seeking treatment or claiming disability for mental, emotional, or psychophysiological distress. This trend should not be discouraged among PG veterans, whose stressors may include experiences from predeployment through combat to reentry to daily living.

Finally, the committee has been concerned that a diagnosis of somatization disorder, PTSD, or other psychiatric illness not be made by default in those cases where a physical diagnosis has not yet been established. Psychiatric diagnoses require specific findings that the disorder is present. Physical illnesses are often accompanied by emotional disturbances or even gross psychopathology, and DSM-IV (APA, 1994) lists some physical illnesses that may present with psychiatric symptoms. A patient whose complaints are not accepted as legitimate over a period of time may also develop symptoms of an adjustment disorder superimposed on the underlying illness, thereby making a basic diagnosis even more difficult.

WOMEN'S HEALTH STUDIES

Approximately 50,000 of the troops deployed to the PG were women. Although women have been present in combat situations during earlier wars (Congress established the Nurse Corps of the Army in 1901 and of the Navy in 1908, and an estimated 5,000–10,000 women served in Vietnam), the number of women in forward combat support positions was uniquely high for the U.S. armed forces during ODS. With the exception of DoD studies conducted in-theater prior to the air war, most studies of the health of PG soldiers include women and men. Findings of these studies are summarized below, and issues related to women's experiences are enumerated along with questions that merit further consideration. The large number of women living in field conditions, working side by side with men, and doing the same work as men under "field expedient conditions" was also unique to this war. These conditions often required work (and exposures) for 16-hour days, 7 days per week, as discussed in Chapter 3.

The health of women veterans is a very important issue in light of projections of a 17% increase in women veterans between 1990 and 2010, when women will represent 6.4% of the total U.S. veteran population (Sorensen and Feild, 1994). In addition, in civilian populations, women's utilization of health services on average exceeds that of men (Nathanson, 1975), so that the types and number of visits and the use of services could be significantly increased. In addition, women's health has been influenced by a social context in which men played the dominant roles. Issues of leadership or management and training raised by having women serve with men in combat roles also may have significant health effects. Health consequences of combat service for women, gender differences in health, and health issues related to men and women serving in combat situations are all considerations in our recommendations for further action.

Health Effects of Combat Service for Women

Given the novel experiences noted above and the large number of women deployed in the PGW, it is important to determine whether there were health problems unique to women. Because limited data are available to answer this question, the topic requires further study. Long-term follow-up of women veterans who served in ODS is needed. Available data suggest a need for a data collection system that will capture important health services (utilization, needs, and issues) in a way that directs immediate action as well as support for future research. It has been well established in civilian populations that women are more willing to report symptoms and use health services more readily than men for symptoms and conditions that affect both sexes (Nathanson, 1975, 1980).

Thus, interpretation of health reports by veterans will require adjustment for gender differences in reporting.

Reports from several studies, including the General Accounting Office (GAO) study of women, confirm that women deployed to the PG could and did accommodate to adverse conditions and, in the short term, did not present with more health and hygiene problems than men (GAO, 1993b). Data presented earlier in this chapter suggest some gender differences in symptom reporting in the DVA registry.

Pregnancy and certain reproductive system problems (including malignancies such as breast, cervical, and ovarian cancer) are problems unique to women. Pregnancy presents a challenge to women's health under any circumstances and may produce unique health problems in combat situations. In the past, the military has forced women to separate because of pregnancy. Indeed, one of six women in the 1985 Veterans Administration survey of female veterans who entered the military in the post-Vietnam era reported being forced to separate from military service for reasons of pregnancy or having children (VA, 1985). To date, there are no published reports or studies concerning women who became pregnant while deployed to the PG or the military management of these situations.

Pierce (1996) identified a stratified sample of 638 women to study 2 years after the PGW and again 2 years later. The sample included active duty, guard, and reserve Air Force components; those deployed to the Gulf versus elsewhere; and those who were parents, as well as nonparents. General physical health, gender-specific health problems, emotional responses to war, and symptoms common in the unexplained illnesses were surveyed with 97% participation of those located ($N = 525$). Women deployed to the PGW reported significantly more general and gender-specific health problems than those deployed elsewhere. Common health problems included skin rash, cough, depression, unintentional weight loss, insomnia, and memory problems. Active duty women reported more general health problems than those in the reserve or guard, despite their younger age. Among those deployed, women who were parents had significantly more health problems. Two years after the PGW, skin rash, depression, unintentional weight loss, and insomnia were significantly more prevalent among those deployed to the Gulf than those not deployed. Four years after deployment, skin rash remained significantly more prevalent among those deployed and cough and memory problems were more prevalent among the deployed. There were no differences in gender-specific health problems 2 years after PGW, but 4 years later, those deployed had a greater prevalence of lumps or cysts in the breasts, abnormal Pap smear results, and headaches. There was a trend for increased prevalence of herpes among those who served in the Gulf for more than 120 days compared with those who served for less than 120 days. Of those deployed to the Gulf, 24% met criteria for PTSD versus 15% of those deployed elsewhere (Pierce, 1996).

A final variety of health problems affecting women includes those producing acute episodes of symptoms (e.g., vaginitis) that indicate special personal support needs. A "field doctrine" for medically appropriate and field expedient approaches to contraception is also needed. This includes ensuring continuity while activated of medication (e.g., oral contraceptives) used prior to deployment.

Gender Differences in Health

Studies of the prevalence of symptoms during deployment in the PGW revealed few differences between women and men of the First Cavalry Division. Men reporting to sick call were more likely to be diagnosed with orthopedic and dermatologic disorders, and women were more likely to be diagnosed with psychiatric and optometric disorders (Hines, 1993). In a cluster study after the occurrence of unexplained illnesses among PGW veterans in Indiana, DeFraites et al. (1992) found that the prevalence of symptoms among men and women reserve troops was similar. Wolfe has reported preliminary results suggesting that acute PTSD symptomatology is significantly associated with a range of self-reported symptoms in women (Wolfe et al., 1994).

Studies of gender differences in PTSD and other symptoms indicate that prior abuse, coupled with exposure to combat stress, may affect women and men differently. The need for prospective longitudinal studies of both women and men was reinforced by results of a study of PTSD symptoms and precombat sexual and physical abuse among Desert Storm veterans who attended a mental health clinic (297 veterans, including 28 women). Women veterans who reported previous abuse had higher Mississippi Scale scores, higher combat-related PTSD and nonspecific PTSD scores, and higher depression scores than those who had not been abused. Precombat-abused male veterans did not differ from the nonabused in PTSD symptoms (Engel et al., 1993).

Still another study of reserve troops found no overall gender differences in PTSD indicators (Mississippi PTSD Scale, Beck Depression Inventory, and SCL-90-R) for noncombat reservists, but gender differences did appear for two specific combat units. The first unit had experienced fatalities and injuries from a SCUD missile attack and the second had morale problems. Thus, data to support gender differences were found only in units in which there had been combat-related trauma or impaired morale (Perconte et al., 1993).

Some investigators have found evidence of anticipatory anxiety about mobilization among Vietnam veteran women who subsequently were diagnosed with PTSD. A small sample of Army reserve nurses who anticipated mobilization during ODS experienced higher levels of anxiety than similar civilian registered nurses. Separation from loved ones and financial concerns were the greatest contributors to anxiety. Detailed and consistent information from army commands reduced anxiety (Wynd and Dziedzicki, 1992). In another study, women who had had PTSD linked to Vietnam service experienced intensification of their distress during ODS regardless of whether they were deployed (Wolfe et al., 1992a).

Aside from these reports, few have examined gender differences in health related to the war. The few reports to date have focused on the development of symptoms and PTSD. In a study of reservists (653 PGW veterans and 259 stateside duty troops), Sutker et al. (1995a) examined the hypothesis that ethnic minority status and female gender were associated with greater psychological distress after war zone duty. All troops were studied within 1 year of return from the Gulf. Women reported more physical or somatic symptoms, including more headaches, lack of energy, cold or flu symptoms, and upset stomach, than men regardless of their deployment status. There were no statistically significant gender differences in depression, anxiety, or anger. Minority men reported more PTSD symptoms than white men. The small numbers of minority women in this study may have limited the ability to detect interactive effects of gender and ethnicity.

Studies examining correlates of symptoms have identified combat stress, sexual harassment and assault, leadership and unit morale, and family care worries as important. One study of women and men immediately after their return from the Gulf demonstrated that both women and men experienced war zone stress related to combat exposure. No significant gender differences in the Laufer combat scores (describing the kinds of combat stressors to which people were exposed) were found, although men's scores were somewhat higher. Results of the more comprehensive ODS expanded checklist found that the three most commonly reported war zone stressors for both genders were formal alert for chemical or biological warfare, receiving incoming fire from large arms, and witnessing death and disfigurement of enemy troops. PTSD scores were higher for women (9% of women and 4% of men scored above 89 on the Mississippi Scale). Women reported more PTSD symptoms and had higher BSI scores than men. These findings suggest that women were more symptomatic during the initial postdeployment phase. Wolfe et al. (1993) suggest that this difference may be attributable to women's socialization; women's reporting symptoms more freely than men; family-related reentry stressors; prior stress, such as sexual or criminal victimization, leaving residual symptoms and greater sensitivity to new stress; and sexual harassment or assault experienced during deployment.

Women with PTSD also reported more physical symptoms than men (Wolfe et al., 1995). This finding suggests that some but not all of the physical symptomatology reported by PGW women vets may be related to PTSD.

Wolfe et al. (1995) found that both men and women reservists reported negative change in physical and psychological health since they returned from the PG and that more women than men reported a change for the worse in both physical and psychological health. More women had evidence of presumptive

PTSD and reported health symptoms in conjunction with PTSD. Headaches, lack of energy, aches or pains, nervousness, tension, insomnia, and depression were endorsed more frequently by women than by men.

Gender differences in needs for support on return home have received little attention, yet it is reasonable to believe that stresses related to separation from home and family affected women and men in different ways. According to preliminary findings by Pierce (1995) among 525 Air Force women who were activated, being a parent was associated with more health problems and depressive symptoms, and this effect was pronounced for women who were deployed in the theater.

Nelson et al. (1996) conducted ethnographic research regarding family support needs associated with mobilization of the National Guard and reserve forces by interviewing 59 military members, family members (including children), commanders, and family support personnel from National Guard and reserve forces; by using participant observation in selected units; and by examining cultural artifacts such as documents, journals, and newspapers. This research involved interviewing in great detail this nonrandomly selected small group of individuals in a very open-ended fashion.

Nelson found that staying connected in an uncertain environment was a universal concern that was exacerbated when units were fragmented. Living with the war was unusual for families who "watched" the war on television as if it were a staged theatrical production. Indeed, military members recounted watching themselves being attacked on television as the attack was occurring and they were putting on protective gear. Fluctuating emotions were common throughout families. Refocusing lives became the major task for the families of those who returned from the Gulf. Family support systems were regarded as helpful but not easily accessed. Moreover, the study revealed a need to train families better to cope with deployment, to improve information transmission, and to support reassimilation after the war. In particular, children needed preparation as did their caretakers. Financial issues were among some of the most difficult for families to resolve (because of the delay in receiving military pay, some families could not buy food). Nelson has indicated that although returning from the Gulf represented a vulnerable period, it also was an opportune time for helping families.

Deployed women whose family issues were well managed may have had reduced anxiety or stress during deployment and reduced familial stress on return from deployment. Further emphasis by commanders of such leadership or management issues for both women and men in combat situations may alleviate some of the problems experienced in-theater and after deployment.

Health Issues Related to Men and Women Serving Together in Combat Situations

In addition to assessing gender differences in health outcomes and exposures, researchers have begun to address the consequences of women and men serving together in combat. Most American military women and men carried themselves through the conflict without major problems, but it remains important to improve the training of both men and women on active duty and in the reserves or National Guard in handling these sensitive issues.

As discussed earlier in this chapter, Wolfe and colleagues have begun to describe women's exposures to stressors such as physical or sexual harassment and assault during deployment. Also, Engel et al. (1993) found that precombat abuse led to higher rates of PTSD symptoms in female PGW veterans and that deployed women with a prior history of abuse had greater PTSD symptomatology than those without a history of abuse. The long-term consequences of abuse prior to deployment, coupled with harassment, discrimination, and abuse during deployment and demobilization, merit further study.

Sexual activity between women and men may eventuate in pregnancy and sexually transmitted disease, both preventable with access to appropriate preventive measures.

Another committee of the IOM (IOM, 1995b) recently reported on research needs related to the health effects of military service on women.

5

Some Hypotheses Regarding Illnesses in Persian Gulf War Veterans

OVERVIEW

In our attempt to investigate comprehensively the health-related consequences of service in the Persian Gulf (PG), we have encountered numerous hypotheses, often provided by independent investigators, that have suggested a wide variety of associations among agents and exposures, circumstances that existed in the Gulf, and adverse clinical outcomes. These hypotheses have had various degrees of plausibility and supporting research. Some investigators brought their work to the attention of the committee. In each case, the material presented by individuals and groups, in person or in documents, was evaluated by the entire committee and considered as we formed our overall impression of the health consequences of service in the Gulf. The many investigations (both federal and private) and the putative causal associations that we evaluated demonstrate the vexing nature of the medical problem presented by what some have referred to as a "Gulf War Syndrome" (GWS), and we refer to as unexplained illnesses (UI).

A précis of many of the hypotheses and much of the supporting evidence that the committee received is provided herein. Most of this material was not solicited. Thus, this list is not intended to be exhaustive or complete, but rather to illustrate the issues that faced both the investigators and the committee. The number and variety of hypotheses call attention to the variety of different types of abnormalities that have been reported and the strong likelihood that no single hypothesis could account for all of these, whether or not the illnesses result from service in the Persian Gulf War (PGW).

The committee has been troubled by news stories about activities to promote the treatment of clinically evident manifestations of UI. These raise ethically troublesome questions about the lack of documented efficacy, and some of these interventions could even prove harmful to individual patients. Finally, since placebo treatment of patients with almost any ailment (psychological or otherwise) will often result in marked improvement in symptoms or even physical signs of disease, well-designed clinical studies must be employed to understand the efficacy of any medical intervention.

CHRONIC FATIGUE SYNDROME

The complaints and signs reported by PGW veterans suggested to some observers the possibility of chronic fatigue syndrome (CFS) as a common diagnostic label. The syndrome is of unknown etiology, occurs worldwide, and is reported to result in significant disability for the patient. Early doubts have not been fully reversed, but there is a growing consensus that CFS may be a valid diagnosis.

This syndrome has been reported in the medical literature for several hundred years (Straus, 1991). Numerous names have been attached to the many symptoms, signs, and laboratory findings identified in investigations of clusters of patients. In 1987 a definition of the syndrome was reached by a consensus development process under the sponsorship of the Centers for Disease Control and Prevention (CDC) (Holmes et al., 1988). Subsequently, similar definitions were published by British (Sharpe et al., 1991) and Australian (Lloyd et al., 1990) epidemiologists. These efforts culminated in 1994 in a combined international case definition that maintained the major components of the 1988 document but reduced the required number of minor symptoms and eliminated all physical findings as a necessary part of the definition (Fukuda et al., 1994). The group settled on the definition given below to facilitate "a more systematic collection of data internationally." An interesting aspect of this syndrome is the reporting by numerous investigators of objective neurologic (Rowe et al., 1995), muscular (Kuratsune et al., 1994), and immunological (Barker et al., 1994) findings. Despite these observations, no common etiology has been identified and not all manifestations are found in each patient. Therefore, such objective evidence is not included in the definition.

This definition (Fukuda et al., 1994) attempts to clarify what fatigue is and includes eight of the most common symptoms of the syndrome. Fatigue, the main CFS symptom, is defined as "self-reported persistent or relapsing fatigue lasting six or more consecutive months," and all other possible medical and psychiatric causes are eliminated. The classification of chronic fatigue syndrome is made when the criteria for severity of fatigue are met and four or more of the following eight symptoms are concurrently present or recurring for 6 or more months of illness not predating fatigue: (1) impaired memory or concentration, (2) sore throat, (3) tender cervical or axillary lymph nodes, (4) muscle pain, (5) multijoint pain without joint swelling or redness, (6) new headaches, (7) nonrefreshing sleep, and (8) postexertion malaise lasting more than 24 hours. Patients who have chronic fatigue but do not meet these criteria are classified as having idiopathic chronic fatigue.

MULTIPLE CHEMICAL SENSITIVITY

As concern over UI has emerged, a condition known as multiple chemical sensitivity (MCS) syndrome has been suggested by several investigators and clinicians as the link between PG veterans' unexplained illness and environmental exposures (Miller, 1994, 1996; Ziem, 1992, 1994). Certain investigators have suggested that PGW veterans who are experiencing multiple symptoms, consistent with the constellation described for MCS, had their disease "induced" by one or more exposure in the Gulf, including pesticides, solvents, drugs, or virtually any of the other agents encountered there. These investigators hypothesize that the subsequent "triggering" of disease occurs after low-level exposures to similar noxious substances, likely becoming manifest after the return home of the affected troops. This process would constitute the "loss of tolerance" as described by Miller (1996).

MCS syndrome has become a diagnosis increasingly assigned to patients with a variety of commonly experienced symptoms attributed to exposure to various environmental chemicals at very low levels (Sparks et al., 1994). Consequently, a working definition of MCS relies on the individual's subjective symptoms of distress, attributed to environmental exposure, rather than on measurable objective evidence. Patients labeled with MCS are clearly distressed and many are functionally disabled. Cullen (1987) defined MCS as "an acquired disorder characterized by recurrent symptoms, referable to multiple organ systems, occurring in response to demonstrable exposure to many chemically unrelated compounds at doses far below those established in the general population to cause harmful effects." He stated that there was no single widely accepted test of physiological function shown to correlate with symptoms. This definition remains the most widely used clinical definition but does not apply to all patients currently diagnosed with MCS.

There are four major views about the etiology of MCS. One view is that MCS is a physical or psychophysiologic reaction to multiple chemicals. A second view is that MCS symptoms may be precipitated by low-level environmental exposures, but the underlying increased sensitivity is initiated primarily by psychologic stress. A third view is that MCS is a misdiagnosis and chemical exposure is not the cause of the symptoms. In this case the symptoms may be due to misdiagnosed physical or psychiatric illness. The fourth view is that MCS is simply a belief system instilled by certain practitioners, the media, or others in society; MCS is, therefore, the manifestation of culturally shaped illness behavior (Sparks et al., 1994). Although there is often a willingness to attribute these symptoms to a primary anxiety disorder, it has been noted that few patients diagnosed as having MCS meet the established criteria for this psychiatric diagnosis.

OXIDATIVE PHOSPHORYLATION DISORDER

McGill (1993, 1995) has suggested that unexplained illnesses are caused by a disorder of the mitochondrial metabolism leading to encephalomyopathy. In this construct, veterans are afflicted with a multisystem, multiorgan disease that has a vast array of secondary complications and can present in a variety of forms and severities. It is presumed to be linked etiologically with poor nutrition combined with increased metabolic demand. Definitive diagnosis of this condition is not straightforward, and there is no current medical consensus concerning the validity of this proposed entity. A series of questionnaires and laboratory tests that focus on neurological and metabolic abnormalities have been proposed as a means of identifying individuals with variations of this syndrome.

DENTAL AMALGAMS

Summers (1994) has proposed that a set of unexplained symptoms in PGW veterans (skin rashes, chronic fatigue, headaches, sore joints, hair loss, irritability, insomnia, diarrhea, and depression) may be related to mercury toxicity occurring as a result of the installation of dental amalgams just prior to or immediately after service in the PGW. This hypothesis asserts that installation of these amalgams resulted in clinically evident elemental mercury toxicity that continues as patients have ongoing exposure to mercury.

Mercury-based dental amalgams have been employed for more than 150 years, and the amalgams used in service personnel are similar to those used in civilian dental practices. It is clear that the placement of dental amalgams results in systemic exposure to mercury (Gross and Harrison, 1989; Summers et al., 1993). It is also clear that significant exposure (e.g., occupational exposure by inhalation) to elemental mercury results in a toxic syndrome with a complex clinical presentation (Wyngaarden et al., 1992). However, the reports of elemental mercury-induced disease available in the literature are associated primarily with inhalation exposures that are very much higher that those associated with amalgam placement (Parkinson, 1992). At the same time, relatively few human studies of adverse effects of amalgams have been done.

Interest in diminishing elemental mercury exposure has resulted in proposals in Sweden, Denmark, and Germany for restrictions on the use of mercury-containing dental amalgams. The U.S. Public Health Service reviewed this issue and concluded that it was inappropriate at that time (1993) to recommend restriction of the use of dental amalgams (DHHS, 1993). Thus, there appears to be consensus in this country that mercury from dental amalgams is unlikely to be the source of significant morbidity. To date, the hypothesis of unexplained symptoms in PGW veterans associated with the recent installation of dental amalgams has not been directly investigated to the best of our knowledge.

BACTERIAL ILLNESS

Persistent streptococcal or other bacteremia has been suggested (Hyman, 1996) as a cause of UI related to service in the Gulf. The suspected bacteremia is proposed to resemble that encountered after dental procedures and is claimed to be diagnosable by using unique microscopic evaluation of the urine, which streptococci enter from the blood via the kidney. No specific exposure in the PG has been suggested to have resulted in infection with the bacterium. This purported bacteremia has been treated with intravenous and oral antibiotics (primarily clindamycin) for extended periods, with undocumented reports of "curing" veterans having unexplained symptoms. To our knowledge, no reports of any study of the risk that this treatment increases the risk of infection by antibiotic-resistant bacteria have been made available. Of note, clindamycin is considered inappropriate for treatment of almost all forms of urinary tract infection. In addition, this antibiotic can produce significant gastrointestinal side effects when used for prolonged periods. The proposer of this hypothesis indicates that he has seen streptococci in urine in civilians for more than 30 years.

Although there have been attempts to initiate a formal study of this putative bacterial syndrome, federal funding for the research has been withheld after review by several groups found the researcher's proposals to be of poor quality. The prevalence of this disorder in otherwise unexposed asymptomatic individuals is unexplored.

MYCOPLASMA AND CHRONIC FATIGUE

Some investigators have hypothesized that a subset of soldiers with unexplained illnesses of a type considered similar to CFS have mycoplasma infections that can be diagnosed if appropriate laboratory tests are available. Nicolson and Nicolson (1995a) have reported on a group of 73 individuals composed primarily of veterans but including some family members (the group is referred to as a nonscientific sample) since mycoplasma infections can be spread by close contact. These individuals with unexplained CFS-like illness were studied for mycoplasma-related DNA detectable in peripheral blood cells, and 55% were found to have evidence of such DNA. These individuals, who were not found to have mycoplasma in the peripheral blood by standard methods, were found to be positive by using a polymerase chain-reaction method targeting DNA in their white blood cells (Nicolson and Nicolson, 1995b). The polymerase chain-reaction method used has not been directly related to pathologic potential or outcome, nor have the results been independently confirmed. No source of mycoplasma infection has been documented, although mention has been made of the potential immunosuppressive effects of inhaled fine sand particulates present in the Gulf region. Nicolson has stated that the preliminary study of this hypothesis did not utilize "a scientific sample" (Nicolson, 1996) and has briefly described studies that have been proposed in collaboration with CDC to further examine this hypothesis. To date the relevance of this finding is unclear.

SKELETAL MUSCLE BIOENERGETICS

This putatively GWS-related clinical entity may share some similarity with disorders of oxidative phosphorylation, also proposed to be causally related to UI (see above). Fishman (1995) examined three veterans with undefined chronic fatigue. Two patients were evaluated by using magnetic resonance imaging, and an additional seven patients are being examined with magnetic resonance spectroscopy for metabolic evaluation of skeletal muscle. The data presented suggest that some sort of abnormalities may be present in muscle oxidative capacity in these veterans, but it is unclear if the abnormalities are related to each other. A brief letter provided to the committee explains that the individuals were referred for evaluation of GWS. The letter did not include demographic or other data on the individuals, such as their age, gender, life-style habits, whether they were taking other medications or had other illness, what branch of the military they were serving in, the sorts of exposure they might have encountered, or how "normal" comparison values were generated for the tests on muscle function. The investigative findings were suggested to potentially contribute to understanding the pathophysiology of fatigue, and no cause for this fatigue was suggested.

SARCOIDOSIS AND LINGUAL ABNORMALITIES

Milner (unpublished) has studied the occurrence of sarcoidosis in PGW veterans self-referred to the Veterans Administration Medical Center (VAMC) in Allen Park, Michigan. This study compared the occurrence of a diagnosis of sarcoidosis in 626 male PGW veterans who were self-referred from 1991 through 1994 with the occurrence of the condition in 9,567 self-referred male veterans who were not deployed to the PG. A total of ten cases of sarcoidosis were diagnosed (all in African Americans): five cases were found in the PGW veterans and five in the non-PGW veterans, resulting in a fifteenfold difference in prevalence. This led to the conclusion that the crude (nonage-adjusted) incidence of sarcoidosis among PGW veterans could be estimated as approximately 800 per 100,000 compared with an estimated 136 per 100,000 in the control group.

The etiology of sarcoidosis is unknown, and this study suggests that further work might be indicated, particularly since there has been some suggestion that sarcoidosis is exposure related. At the same time, the prevalence reported in this study seems unlikely to account for a significant portion of illness in PGW veterans.

Other studies at the same VAMC have suggested that there is a "toxic exposure sign" associated with ill health related to service in the Gulf. Milner and Plezia (1995) have reported that 33% of the PG veterans they examined had lingual papillitis as well as lingual and buccal hairy striae. The lingual findings are reported as painless multiple erythematous papular elevations along the anterodorsal aspect of the tongue, which appeared to be inflamed hypertrophic filiform papillae. These veterans were noted to have multiple linear inflamed areas along the cheek and occasionally along the dorsolateral surface of the tongue. The authors suggest that the findings may serve as an initial sign that the patient is suffering multisystem effects of toxic exposure.

As a biological model, Milner and colleagues (unpublished) have suggested that the unexplained illness associated with PGW service is the result of an immunopathologic picture of immunosuppression. The immunosuppression has, in this model, resulted in type 1, type 2, type 3, and type 4 hypersensitivity reactions. These reactions, again in this model, are putatively related to low-dose, repetitive exposure to "extracellular antigens"; exposure to intracellular antigens presented at high dose; and finally, exposure to "reactivated viral infections." In this fashion, multiple-system disease with many secondary manifestations can be seen as the natural outcome of a single pathologic entity.

To date, no confirmatory studies of these hypotheses have been investigated. Information on sarcoidosis diagnoses in other geographic locations is lacking, and as yet, the "toxic exposure sign" has not been noted by other investigators.

BRAINSTEM DYSREGULATION SYNDROME

One investigator has undertaken a case investigation of 10 PGW veterans who reported heat intolerance or photophobia, autonomic instability with headaches, and the presence of motor abnormalities, exaggerated startle response to noise, or decreased sense of taste (Baumzweiger, 1996). Based on detailed investigation of these 10 cases and his general observations of similar symptoms in nonveterans, the investigator has developed a hypothesis of a syndrome experienced by PGW veterans that is called the "Two-Hit Brainstem Syndrome." The hypothesis suggests that two "insults" to the brainstem, one early in life and one later (e.g., while in the Gulf region), could produce a polysymptomatic illness. The combined result is loss of control over the T-cell lymphocyte receptor, with resulting confrontation between the attentional and immune systems. The consequence is increasingly poor response to brainstem-related adaptive mechanisms. No testable specification of this hypothesis has been presented and no study protocol has been reviewed by the committee.

MICROSPORIDIA INFECTION

One VAMC investigator examined the stool of PGW veterans to search for protozoal infections using histochemical staining techniques (Blanck, 1996). Based on the results of these tests and the size characteristics of bodies noted in the stools from 133 of the 143 individuals tested, the investigator suggested that microsporidia infection might be related to service in the PGW. Similar bodies were reported in individuals at the same location who were diagnosed with AIDS, cancer, or chronic steroid therapy. Intensive follow-up investigation of these findings was undertaken by using specimens from these individuals and from PGW veterans at other locations. The specimens were examined by experts in protozoal disease using electron microscopy, immunofluorescence, and special staining techniques. No microsporidia were identified. One expert consulted suggested that the bodies originally noted had been yeast. An investigation of stool specimens collected in one case-control study of PGW veterans revealed no positive stool specimens.

ORGANOPHOSPHATE-INDUCED DELAYED NEUROTOXICITY

The multiplicity of symptoms involved in the PGW-related unexplained illnesses have led a group of investigators to survey the 24th Reserve Naval Seabee Battalion (Haley, 1995). Seven hundred and twenty individuals were mailed the survey and approximately one-third participated. Of this one-third, there was a cluster of individuals who reported symptoms consistent with damage of the central and peripheral nervous systems. Based on this information, the investigators have proposed that the unexplained illnesses are related to delayed toxicity, such as has been described with organophosphate exposure.

Unpublished reports of the results of this study have indicated that there may be some evidence of delayed neurotoxicity associated with symptoms in veterans. As of May 1996, no peer-reviewed report of this small study was available for the committee. While it may serve as an example for hypothesis generation, the study has significant problems, including small sample size, response, possible selection bias, and recall bias. There are no definite exposure measurements in the study group, and multiple hypotheses have been tested in conducting the study.

CHEMICALLY INDUCED PORPHYRIA

It has been suggested that some of the unexplained symptoms reported by PGW veterans are similar to those present in individuals with chemically induced porphyrias (Donnay, 1994). Those proposing this hypothesis indicate a concern that pesticide exposures in the Gulf region may have caused such symptoms, which include photosensitivity to sunlight and occasional dark-brown to red-colored urine. These findings are suggested to be similar to those in individuals who are reported to have MCS syndrome. No formal proposal of a study of this hypothesis was received by the committee.

FIBROMYALGIA

Unexplained illnesses that have been seen in veterans have been said to be strikingly similar to the condition known as fibromyalgia. The diagnosis of fibromyalgia is based on symptoms presented by the patient and one symptom-related physical finding: namely, at any of multiple sites of the body, pinching or pressure by a probing finger induces unexpected withdrawal or exclamations of pain. This discriminating criterion is a major diagnostic finding that, along with widespread musculoskeletal pain, is part of the classification proposed in 1990 by the American College of Rheumatology (Wolfe et al., 1990).

The nature and etiology of fibromyalgia remain elusive. Patients diagnosed with fibromyalgia often also have symptoms that overlap those described for MCS and CFS. Fatigue can be the presenting complaint, as can weakness, sleep disturbance, cognitive complaints, arthralgia, or myalgia. There has been speculation that central nervous system hyperactivity, associated with an increase in excitatory neuropeptides or a decrease in inhibitory neurotransmitters (e.g., serotonin), leads to many of these symptoms. Thus, this cascade is associated with increased sensitivity to pain, autonomic dysregulation, and neuroendocrine disturbances.

Although there has been little systematic study of fibromyalgia in veterans, the symptom complex has been noted in some veterans to parallel that reported for UI. This has led to speculation that some of the unexplained illnesses may have an fibromyalgia-like character. However, no definite exposure or experience has yet been linked to this entity; thus, its possible relationship to PGW service remains unclear.

SOMATIZATION DISORDER

Unexplained illnesses have also been compared with a polysymptomatic condition termed somatization disorder. This entity has its clinical onset prior to age 30, extends over a period of years, and is characterized by a combination of pain with gastrointestinal, sexual, and pseudoneurological symptoms (APA,

1994). The symptoms cause clinically significant distress or impairment in social, occupational, or other areas of functioning. In contrast to factitious disorders or "malingering," the physical symptoms in this disorder are not under voluntary control.

An essential feature of somatization disorder is a pattern of recurring multiple somatic complaints that cannot be fully explained by any known general condition or by the result of exposure to any known substance. Somatization associated with a companion general medical condition results in physical complaints in excess of those expected from evaluation of the patient. Individuals with this disorder usually describe their complaints in colorful, exaggerated terms, but factual information is often lacking.

In a presentation to the committee, Barsky (1995) discussed four major influences in the reporting of symptoms. Cognition influences are the first important factor in symptom reporting; that is, when people notice symptoms, they try to attribute or make hypotheses that might explain their symptoms. Symptoms attributed to disease are generally perceived as more intense than symptoms that are dismissed. Another important factor in reporting symptoms is the context of what is being perceived. The occurrence of the symptom and people's experiences of a symptom will influence how it is reported. A third factor is attention as an amplifier of a symptom. Paying attention to a symptom will intensify it, and to some extent, the symptom can be "infectious." The fourth factor influencing symptom reporting is mood, with anxiety and depression being important influences and amplifiers of symptoms.

SUMMARY

The committee found these descriptions of ongoing work interesting for a variety of reasons. First, their diverse nature provides additional compelling evidence that no one disease entity will likely be adequate to resolve the understanding of all unexplained illnesses in PG veterans. Second, these ideas, hypotheses, and investigations also serve as testimony to the efforts of many health professionals who strive to find avenues, overlooked by others, that might lead to new understanding of these illnesses and result in amelioration of the suffering that has occurred and continues to be reported. Third, although these approaches have varying merit and the investigators are dedicated to solving the problem, we are not optimistic that any are sufficiently well substantiated to offer much hope of important answers or relief for significant numbers of ailing American veterans. Hypotheses can be tested in research that has undergone scientific review by one's peers and been submitted for publication in a peer-reviewed journal for the scientific community as a whole to evaluate.

Finally, although the committee has not identified an explanation for the unexplained illnesses in PG veterans, we do not doubt that many individuals reporting such illness are seriously affected. We also recognize that many illnesses in the population at large lack explanation according to current medical understanding and also require an open mind. Continuing efforts to explore all possible avenues to increase our knowledge of such illnesses, and to reduce suffering and disability, are certainly indicated. The fact that work of the tentative nature summarized here continues 6 years after cessation of the PGW underscores the importance of taking seriously the reports of ill health among active and returning troops. Those involved in future conflicts must anticipate the need to integrate into Defense Department and Department of Veterans Affairs planning at all stages high-quality research on the health consequences of combat and of deployments to hostile environments.

6

Information Systems

OVERVIEW

The single most troublesome problem encountered in attempts to conduct epidemiologic studies of illnesses among Persian Gulf War (PGW) veterans has been the inability to retrieve information on medical care events such as hospitalizations, outpatient visits, and diagnoses and treatments from Department of Defense (DoD) and Department of Veterans Affairs (DVA) medical records in a uniform and systematic manner. Lack of uniform and retrievable medical information concerning reserve, National Guard, active, and separated forces has greatly inhibited systematic analysis of the health effects of mobilization. DoD and DVA have different and only partially automated inpatient hospital record systems. Neither DoD nor DVA has automated outpatient record keeping, although the committee has recently learned that a database with outpatient records will be available in the near future from DVA. Current systems are fragmented, disorganized, incomplete, and therefore poorly suited to support epidemiologic and health outcomes studies.

As an interim measure to obtain information about exposures, health, and medical care among PGW veterans, DoD and DVA established four independent programs: the DVA Persian Gulf Health Registry (PGHR), DoD Comprehensive Clinical Evaluation Program (CCEP), DoD Troop Exposure Assessment Model (TEAM), and DoD Registry of Unit Locations (RUL).

The committee finds that the PGHR and CCEP are useful for clinical evaluation of the health problems of PGW veterans but cannot be utilized for research because they include only self-selected individuals who volunteer to participate in these programs. TEAM and RUL also will have limited utility for epidemiologic studies since they provide information at the unit level rather than at the individual level.

Whereas no system of medical record keeping can or should be designed to provide the information needed to address every unanticipated issue regarding the health consequences of either military service in general or a specific military conflict, health information systems can be established to facilitate epidemiologic studies of such service. The committee has identified several changes in health information systems for military personnel that will enhance the capability of the military to evaluate the health consequences of future deployments and service. These include creation of a uniform medical record (UMR), including data from civilian providers; full implementation of the Defense Medical Epidemiological Database (DMED) system; and completion of the Army's Patient Accounting and Reporting Real-Time Tracking System (PARRTS), including expansion to the other branches of service.

Medical care and health surveillance (for persons who may need medical attention now) and epidemiologic evaluation of potential threats to the health of service personnel (for research to prevent future problems) will be greatly strengthened by the development of a system that provides access to the entire medical history of each member of the armed services and facilitates linkage to other sources of data. Such a system would provide substantial benefits to the service member and veteran, to future service persons whose health will be better protected, and to DoD or any agency that needs healthy personnel.

As far back as World War I, and perhaps antiquity, every war has left a proportion of service personnel and veterans with serious medical complaints that are not explainable on the basis of known health hazards or identified physical illnesses. This pattern is so consistent, and the health problems are so important, that databases and health information systems should be designed and implemented now to deal with and mitigate similar problems that are likely to arise in future conflicts.

This chapter addresses the committee's charge to "assess the effectiveness of actions taken by the Secretary of Veterans Affairs and the Secretary of Defense to collect and maintain information that is potentially useful for assessing the health consequences of . . . military service" and to "make recommendations on means of improving the collection and maintenance of such information" (see Appendixes A, B). The chapter focuses on two categories of health and exposure information systems: (1) those established in response to health concerns related to service in the PGW and (2) those developed to improve the future capability to evaluate military-service-related health issues.

Several systems exist for collecting health and exposure information. Some are relevant to clinical evaluations, others are relevant to research, and some are relevant to both. Not all of these information systems are appropriate for use in research activities, nor do they have to be. Some of these systems, such as inpatient hospitalization data, were available at the time of the PGW; others, such as the PGHR, were established shortly thereafter; still others, such as PARRTS, have been developed or extended since the PGW. Some of these systems will be useful for collecting data that strengthen future military health preparedness to address research questions.

CRITERIA FOR A RESEARCH-ORIENTED HEALTH INFORMATION SYSTEM

Information systems should include data items that are selected to meet a clearly articulated purpose. A clear statement of objectives for an information system is essential to selecting appropriate and necessary data items for inclusion; determining the level of detail required; and assessing data completeness, accuracy, and utility.

If information systems for DoD and DVA are to support the delivery of high-quality medical care during mobilization and the evaluation of health consequences associated with the conflict, information should be collected for each individual or for well-defined subpopulations and should include at least the following:

1. a list of all individuals participating in activities related to the conflict, to establish the population at risk;
2. complete and accurate information pertaining to the experiences, exposures, and environment of the individuals comprising the population at risk;
3. health experiences prior to mobilization, during mobilization, and after the conflict; and
4. complete and accurate data on personal risk factors for adverse health outcomes and prior health history.

Health information systems should be complete, accurate, cost-effective, and readily usable for practical applications. Therefore, each data item should clearly support the stated objectives of the information system, provide useful insight into health concerns within acceptable time frames, and facilitate decision making for prevention and health care programs. Continual evaluation is essential.

It is not possible to design and implement an information system that can anticipate every question of current or future concern, but systems can be developed to maximize the opportunity to detect trends, define areas of concern, direct corrective actions, and identify needs for supplementary data collection. Here we discuss systems developed specifically to address PGW issues and systems being developed to meet future needs for improved military health information systems.

Appendix G includes a partial listing of existing databases that could provide information for a Medical Health Surveillance System (MHSS) for the armed forces and others that may be useful sources of supplementary information. The large number of existing databases are administered independently and are rarely linked to each other, which highlights the problems of fragmentation and disorganization.

PERSIAN GULF WAR HEALTH INFORMATION SYSTEMS

Several information systems have been developed in response to concerns about the health consequences of the PGW. Those designed to obtain health information include DVA's PGHR and DoD's CCEP. Other systems are designed to obtain exposure information, including TEAM and RUL.

The PGHR includes active duty, retired, reserve, and National Guard veterans of the PGW who are self-referred to obtain a medical examination and appropriate follow-up and to provide registry information. Recently, the committee has learned that provisions are being made to include spouses and offspring of PG veterans in this database. The PGHR contains identifying and demographic information, history of tobacco use, exposure to selected potentially hazardous substances and experiences, diagnosed diseases and conditions, and self-reported symptoms (DVA, 1995b). The CCEP includes self-referred individuals who are experiencing illnesses that may be related to their service in the PGW and are currently on active duty. Eligible family members are also examined. This program was designed to evaluate and treat the health problems of these individuals. Therefore, data contained in this system include demographic and identifying information, medical history data, self-reported symptoms, physical examination data, laboratory test results, diagnostic data, reported workdays lost, and family member data (DoD, 1996; IOM, 1996).

Other information systems were designed to gather or use exposure data. TEAM was presented to the committee as including National Oceanic and Atmospheric Administration (NOAA) models for the entire period of the oil well fires, troop unit locations and movement data, satellite imagery to determine the daily geographic extent of oil fire plumes, U.S. Army Center for Health Promotion and Preventive Medicine (USACHPPM) air pollution data, and other relevant exposure and toxicologic information when and if it becomes available. Recently, the committee learned that data on some individuals who had received the botulinum toxoid or the anthrax vaccine have been included in the database. If TEAM is to be useful for research, it must contain accurate environmental measurements, plausible computer estimates for the time periods of greatest concern, and the ability to link these data systems to each other.

One component of TEAM is RUL, which is an example of a geographical information system (GIS). RUL establishes the latitude and longitude of each military unit at the company level from January 15, 1991, to the date that unit left the Gulf region. TEAM therefore excludes some troops involved in Operation Desert Shield who left the Gulf prior to January 15, 1991. Locations will be recorded for the unit rather than the individual soldier. For example, a time series of geographic locations of troop units might be useful to distinguish between units that were in the vicinity of Kuwait oil well fires and units that were in the area but not downwind from the plume. These data could be a useful resource for general exposure information for units of PGW troops, but they are likely to be subject to misclassification of exposures at the individual level, particularly for individuals with assignments out of their units for particular segments of time.

Some investigators hope to use the RUL database to assess other exposures, such as proximity to depleted uranium (DU) weapons during tank battles. Such a population might have greater potential exposure to DU than other troop units. Investigating possible disease clusters is another potential use of this database—for example, studying diseases or symptoms among units closest to damaged Iraqi chemical weapons depots.

Unit location data will be linked to models of oil well fire location, oil fire plume location, and air pollution data collected by the Army beginning in May 1991. Plans include the development of individual exposure information matrices. Risk values for putative carcinogenic and noncarcinogenic exposures will be determined from sampled as well as modeled grid data. Risk information is to be provided to individual veterans, but this step should be carefully planned and should include explanations of the limitations of interpolating unit data to individuals.

Unit-level data are "ecologic" in nature because each person in a given unit will be assigned the average or aggregate exposure for the entire unit. With ecologic data, information about the joint distribution of exposure and health outcome at the individual level is unknown. This can give rise to the "ecologic fallacy," in which the true exposure-response relationship at the individual level is biased by the grouping of data and possibly by uncontrolled confounding at the individual level. This bias could result in either overestimating or underestimating the risk being considered.

Other limitations affect one-time ecologic summaries of environmental conditions such as oil fire plumes. Exposures that have varying intensity or are characterized by a "pulsing" or short duration of exposure may be inadequately measured. Late placement of health professionals to document these changing conditions in-theater has probably led to mismeasurement of exposures; this may be especially serious for troops or units with the highest levels of exposure.

Inadequate data will severely limit the ability of analyses to establish a connection between a service-related exposure and health outcomes or to demonstrate a dose-response relationship. Merely confirming the presence of a potential hazard in the combat environment does not indicate whether the exposure itself caused the adverse effect or whether there was a level of exposure below which no adverse effect occurred. These questions must be assessed accurately to respond to service members' questions and to evaluate the effectiveness of current preventive medicine practice and of protective equipment and programs.

HEALTH INFORMATION SYSTEMS FOR THE FUTURE

New information systems are being planned and developed to improve military readiness to respond to future health concerns of military service and deployments. These include the UMR, DMED, and Army PARRTS.

The committee has identified several changes in systems and practices for collection of information on the health and service-related exposures of military personnel that will increase the ability of the military services to pursue epidemiologic investigations and health outcomes studies. These changes will increase the capacity of the services to evaluate the efficacy of mobilization-supporting health services, including prevention programs; premobilization, mobilization, and demobilization services; and routine military medical care.

The most important of the proposed changes is the creation of a uniform, continuous, and retrievable medical record. The UMR system should include a minimal data set for all service personnel, encompassing personal and demographic descriptions; health- and service-related exposures; illnesses, injuries, and medical conditions that occur during military service; hazardous and potentially hazardous exposures, job assignments, and locations throughout military service; and periods on temporary duty assignment for training and during deployment for military action, particularly to overseas locations. It also should include information about medical contacts that occur after military discharge through the DVA or other government medical providers and, wherever possible, private providers.

This information should be collected according to standardized procedures and maintained in a computer-accessible format. The primary value of a uniform and centralized record system used by all military services will be an improvement in the health protection and treatment of individuals. Another important benefit will be the support of epidemiologic investigations. A UMR would facilitate selection of appropriate comparison groups as well as linkage to civilian data sources, such as cancer registries, mortality files, and birth defects registries for health outcomes assessment. A UMR also could facilitate follow-up and follow-back by linkage with such electronic data sources as the Health

Care Financing Administration, the National Death Index, and other data files. These sources are utilized for vital status follow-up in longitudinal studies. Although attractive scientifically, follow-up methods, linkages, and information collected require careful attention to informed consent and privacy protection.

A UMR would solve certain problems in the current medical information systems as well. Most current medical information is in the traditional paper format. Electronic data are limited primarily to hospital inpatient discharge summaries, utilizing international diagnostic codes for predominant medical conditions and the more common medical procedures. Information from mobilization stations and mobile field medical facilities is most likely to be incomplete and to be separated from other military medical records. A single computerized record that follows each individual throughout all facilities would solve many of these problems. Furthermore, such a UMR system would eliminate the need to establish conflict-specific registries for current and future deployments.

In the construction of the UMR and related databases and their application to military health issues, care must be taken to safeguard the privacy and confidentiality of military personnel and their family members encompassed by these systems.

The committee has identified three aspects of current policies and practices that must be modified to support the completion and implementation of integration of medical record systems and their coordination with civilian medical records. The first is the policy of assigning separate responsibility to each military service for the medical records of active personnel and separate responsibility to DVA for the medical records of veterans in its facilities. Second, medical records established and maintained by the reserves and National Guard are kept separate from each of the above and are not routinely linked. As a result of these practices, the content of the medical record differs among medical services. Third, data recorded by the reserves, National Guard, DVA, and DoD are not linked to data from civilian physicians and facilities. Therefore, one cannot obtain a comprehensive profile of the health of service personnel discharged from active duty.

The committee concludes that the branches of the military service, the reserve and National Guard organizations, and the DVA must work together in the development of standardized and uniformly applied practices regarding the collection, recording, and maintenance of service health records. Medical care of the individual, the efficiency and effectiveness of the medical care system, health surveillance, and epidemiologic evaluation of potential threats to the health of service personnel will be greatly strengthened by the development of a system that provides access to the entire medical history of each member of the armed services.

The committee is mindful of the need for meticulous attention to many difficulties that will arise in the last step of this proposed data system—the linkage to civilian sources. Those difficulties will include concerns about privacy and confidentiality, costs imposed on the provider of the information (individually small perhaps, but large in the aggregate), barriers to integrating information from civilian sources that is not provided in a UMR format, the need for very rapid response regarding individual medical problems, and the sheer size of the proposed system. We believe that these problems can be solved, but solutions will take time. Delay in integrating data from the civilian sector must not be allowed to retard progress in integrating data from all segments of the military.

The committee is encouraged that efforts are being made toward unifying medical records among the service branches, and computerizing parts of this record in a uniform way is being discussed. It is understandable that each service will have aspects of the medical record that are specific to its mission; however, uniform collection of core data items is important.

The complexity of medical information systems and the problems encountered in obtaining such data are exacerbated when investigations focus upon reproductive outcomes. Therefore, problems related to health studies in this area highlight issues critical for developing a military medical information system.

Discharge summaries, records of infant births, and records of congenital malformations recognized at the time of a newborn's discharge from the hospital are collected in a standardized manner throughout DoD medical treatment facilities worldwide. However, only limited data are available from insurance records such as CHAMPUS (Civilian Health and Medical Program of the Uniformed Services—a civilian community-managed care plan for DoD beneficiaries) or from TRICARE (regionalized tri-service health care system). These data may be useful for studying the effects of service on late-gestational pregnancy losses, prematurity, birth weight, and major malformations identifiable within the first days of life. Data are less likely to be available for infertility, pregnancy loss prior to the third trimester, delayed growth and development of offspring, or any condition dealt with by civilian health care providers. The committee has been told that service members on active duty often choose to obtain reproductive care from civilian sources, thus highlighting the need for linkage of this important area of military medical research with civilian medical records.

Although a uniform medical record would substantially strengthen the ability of the military services to evaluate the health of service personnel and the efficacy of military health programs and doctrine, it cannot provide all of the information that might be needed to respond to unanticipated health problems arising after a deployment. Several supplementary databases are described below.

The committee has heard presentations on the DMED system under development by the three services and the DVA. This system will contain standardized data elements from each service's epidemiologic database, including demographic data (sex, race, ethnicity, date of birth, marital status, education), personnel data (personal identification number, rank, duty station, unit identification code, unit zip code, DoD occupation group, length of service, dates of active service), and medical events (hospitalization dates, disposition, up to eight diagnoses and eight procedures, cause of injury, sick days per episode, medical treatment facility, autopsy). Future expansion of DMED may include deployment data, medical readiness data (vaccinations, examination status), temporary duty stations, reserve and National Guard data, and outpatient data.

Many important research investigations could be undertaken with such information. The fully developed system will, however, have other research capabilities. First, it can be used as an index to persons who have specific features, for example, all those who may have had military occupational exposure to some solvent or all those who have developed some specific form of cancer. Such persons can then be studied in greater depth from the original health records, personal interviews, or other information sources. Second, a complete listing can be used as a "sampling frame" for detailed study of a random sample of persons with specific characteristics, such as a sample of all those who served in the PGW. This may be critical when the intensity of analysis precludes study of all persons who have specific features (e.g., the 697,000 who served in the PGW).

The committee believes that mechanisms should be established to collect more extensive data during periods of deployment and combat. A presentation and demonstration to the committee of the Army's PARRTS indicated that significant efforts have been made to collect in-theater hospitalization data. Inclusion of information from other services and casualties and addition of information on ambulatory care will strengthen the ability of this system to provide real-time data on medical conditions in-theater. PARRTS demonstrates that the Army has initiated real-time electronic submission of data describing health conditions that may compromise the success of a mission and events that may reflect a breakdown in the prevention of illness. These data will have to be linked to individual health information in other databases or in the UMR to be of value beyond the reporting of aggregate combat field hospitalizations. A central group of civilian experts, military specialists, and major operational commanders should review and evaluate the program periodically as one means to advance its mission.

The current surveillance of reportable illnesses and the publication of the *Medical Surveillance Monthly Report* by the Army provide timely data for the entire Army, not just the deployed forces. Similarly, it is important that real-time data collection be monitored to document the numbers of key adverse health effects and the characteristics of the population from which they derive. Medical profiles should be updated periodically to reflect current experiences.

For each military operation, prior or concurrent identification of plausible infectious threats or environmental hazards to health will assist in determining what additional data should be collected for specific in-theater exposures. Additional information needed will depend on geographic area, endemic diseases, nature of the conflict, expected duration and intensity of exposures, and perhaps other factors specific to the conflict. Forward planning for a range of future conflicts will be required, along with ongoing revision during mobilization and deployment, during the conflict itself, and during the postwar period.

Establishment by the Army of the Theater Area Medical Laboratory (TAML) for the purposes of identifying and evaluating medical problems and conducting studies during deployments will improve the capability to investigate potential health problems and disease outbreaks while troops are still in the field. However, the success of this concept in the future will depend on the commander's support and commitment to utilize the unit early in deployment. The expertise in epidemiology and the clinical and laboratory diagnostic capabilities offered by TAML could provide immediate and useful guidance and capability to collect information in the field when problems or unusual exposures are identified.

In combat situations, military success is, of course, all important. Our recommendations in no way suggest or endorse compromising the military mission for the purpose of improving health data collection. Questions about possible acute or delayed health effects of military service must not interfere with operational activities in any way that could degrade effectiveness in successfully fulfilling the primary military mission. Rather, there should be prior and concurrent review and planning by experts who understand both the military imperatives and the health consequences of service to establish the appropriate mechanisms to collect these data. Two examples from the PGW where improvements in data maintenance would have been valuable are the preservation of predeployment immunization records and a more full, informative, and nonthreatening health assessment at the time of demobilization.

CONCLUSIONS

The purposes of medical records and research records differ, but there is great benefit in collecting as much information as possible in a structured format. This structure will reduce data errors, be compatible with computerized clinical data systems, and be available for research studies. A medical record system for patient care should be constructed with major input from physicians, nurses, and administrators and should be oriented largely toward the care of the individual patient. There is a need for a detailed record of personal, family, and medical history; symptoms at the time the patient is first seen and later; physical findings and how they change; results of each laboratory test and radiological procedure; detailed records of findings at surgery and from pathology examination; reasons for and results of specialist referrals; daily or even hourly nurses' notes; and condition at discharge, with copies of any instructions provided to the patient regarding activity level, drugs, return visits, etc. Considerable information must be in free-form text, but much can be collected in a structured format.

Although patient care data should be collected in as structured a format as possible, the requirements of research studies are somewhat more stringent. A research protocol generally requires additional structure. For example, the investigator may need to collect the same data items for each patient in the same way at the same time point in the medical process. Requirements for precision of observations may also be more rigorous (e.g., special devices and techniques to measure liver function with more precision than is needed for clinical care), and some observations may have to be made with increased frequency. Thus, data items of research interest tend to be more numerous, more precise, and more patterned than those for patient care only. Importantly, most of the text in a clinical record will be of little value to the researcher in that format, although it may have a very important role in helping to understand a complicated medical situation and in the completion and accurate coding of structured items. Computerizing the entire medical record may also reduce the cost of research that utilizes the data, since access to such information will be more efficient.

Because of the need for meticulous attention to research needs for specific data in a sometimes unavoidably chaotic medical setting, investigators often find that they must take the lead in screening and securing the data they require, and the data must be available in their laboratories or offices. However, a combined system of records for patient care and research will be increasingly feasible, and the collection of structured data should be maximized.

The committee considers these four steps—(1) the development of a uniform medical record, (2) the improvement of data collection on exposures and health status of deployed service personnel, (3) the provision of supplementary data on occupational and environmental exposures, and (4) the inclusion of early detection medical teams during major deployments—to be important elements of an MHSS that would increase the nation's capacity to address questions about the acute and chronic health consequences of deployments of U.S. military service personnel.

In summary, an MHSS would establish the capacity to respond to questions such as the following:

1. What are the baseline personal characteristics and medical status of military service personnel? To what extent are these baseline or preexisting characteristics correlated with the risk of future illnesses and adverse health conditions? Is any correlation likely to be one of cause and effect?

2. For each activity in, or in support of, combat-related military duty, what assignments and exposures are potentially hazardous to health? How great is the hazard?

3. What is the incidence of illnesses, injuries, and medical conditions occurring during routine active military duty?

4. What incident illnesses, injuries, and medical conditions occur during combat-related military duty? Does their frequency or severity change because of specific deployment activities?

5. What hazardous exposures and assignments experienced during active military duty can be linked to specific health outcomes, particularly military-unique exposures or exposure conditions that are significantly different from civilian settings?

6. What preventive measures can be taken prior to or during known exposures to specific hazardous substances or conditions? Are important positive synergies or adverse interactions anticipated among the multiple prevention approaches employed (multiple vaccines, chemopreventives, uniform repellents, area spraying, etc.)?

The development of an MHSS should focus on several issues. Data quality should reflect attention to case and item definitions and ease of input. Data systems should serve a shared purpose among all participating services, agencies (the DoD, DVA, Department of Health and Human Services, Environmental Protection Agency, etc.), and components (active, reserve, and National Guard troops). A lead agency should be identified as the government's proponent and authority for maintaining the MHSS.

Recent military deployments have raised questions of service-connected adverse health effects of delayed onset. These often will be identified and treated in DVA or civilian settings after active military demobilization. As a result, it will be extremely important for DoD to ensure that active military health data systems facilitate efforts to address questions that arise months or years after personnel leave active service or that occur among their family members. Such a proposal would require a research capability and supporting health information system that do not exist today in either DoD or DVA. Cooperation of agencies within the government toward this objective is essential to establishment of an effective MHSS.

Questions about the frequency of health events also occur independently of deployment. Therefore, national data systems maintained by government agencies such as the Department of Health and Human Services or the Centers for Disease Control and Prevention should be analyzed to obtain baseline or comparison data for referent populations. Participation and oversight of experts external to the government will increase the operational effectiveness of such health information systems.

Any impediment to health care access by service members decreases the ability of health information system to recognize that health events are occurring and to assess their service-connectedness in a timely manner. Such obstacles to access to health care after the PGW resulted in amplification of concern, exaggerated community and political response, and well-intended but occasionally unwise and potentially uninformative government-funded activities, as described throughout this report.

Information systems developed immediately after the PGW are limited in scope and disconnected from each other. Systems under development to ensure future medical readiness and to enhance epidemiologic capabilities have great potential for producing a seamless medical record that can be linked to other information systems, and thus meet the important military medical objectives of prevention, providing effective and appropriate medical care, and facilitating epidemiologic research.

References

Abou-Donia MB, Lapadula DM. 1990. Mechanisms of organophosphorus ester-induced delayed neurotoxicity: Type I and type II. Annual Review of Pharmacology and Toxicology 30:405–440.

Abou-Donia MB, Wilmarth KR, Jensen KF, Oehme FW, Kurt TL. 1996. Neurotoxicity resulting from coexposure to pyridostigmine bromide, DEET, and permethrin: Implications of Gulf War chemical exposures. Journal of Toxicology and Environmental Health 48:35–56.

AFIP (Armed Forces Institute of Pathology). 1994. Draft metal analysis for the 11ACR.

Allen SN, Lundberg KJ, Jensen J, Magill J, Aikins T, Hembury M. 1991. Operation Desert Storm: Activation, Deployment and Re-integration Experiences of VA Medical Center Employees. VA Medical Center, Salt Lake City, Utah.

APA (American Psychiatric Association). 1987. DSM-III-R: Diagnostic and Statistical Manual of Mental Disorders. 3rd ed. Washington, D.C.: APA.

APA. 1994. DSM-IV: Diagnostic and Statistical Manual of Mental Disorders. 4th ed. Washington, D.C.: APA.

Arnold SF, Klotz DM, Collins BM, Vonier PM, Guillette LJ Jr., McLachlan JA. 1996. Synergistic activation of estrogen receptor with combinations of environmental chemicals. Science 272:1489–1492.

Baker D, Campbell N, Dyrenforth S, Grace M, Koruna W, Lieneck M, Welch R. 1992. Operation Desert Storm outreach program. Pp. 109–130 in Returning Persian Gulf

Troops: First Year Findings. West Haven, Conn.: VA Northeast Program Evaluation Center.

Barker E, Fujimura SF, Fadem MB, Landay AL, Levy JA. 1994. Immunological abnormalities associated with chronic fatigue syndrome. Clinical Infectious Diseases 18(Suppl 1):S136–S141.

Barsky A. 1995. Somatization Disorders. Presentation to the IOM Committee to Review Health Consequences of Service During the Persian Gulf War, Washington, D.C., May 1995.

Baumzweiger WE. 1996. Brainstem dysregulation syndrome: A neuropsychiatric symptom complex caused by multiple sequential insults to immune-attentional brainstem function as seen in case studies of Gulf War veterans and environmentally compromised disability applicants in Los Angeles, Calif. Presentation to the IOM Committee to Review Health Consequences of Service During the Persian Gulf War. Irvine, Calif., January 1996.

Bender AP, Williams AN, Johnson RA, Jagger HG. 1990. Appropriate public health responses to clusters: The art of being responsibly responsive. American Journal of Epidemiology 132(Suppl 1):S48–S52.

Berg W. 1994. Post-Persian Gulf Medical Findings: Naval Mobile Construction Battalion 24. Presentation to NIH Technology Assessment Workshop Panel on the Persian Gulf Experience and Health, Bethesda, Md., April 1994.

Bernstein JA, Herd ZA, Bernstein DI, Korbee L, Bernstein IL. 1993. Evaluation and treatment of localized vaginal immunoglobulin E-mediated hypersensitivity to human seminal plasma. Obstetrics and Gynecology 82:667–673.

Berté, SB. 1994. Repellents for the soldier. Army Research, Development, and Acquisition Bulletin July/August:30–32.

Blanck RR. 1996. Memorandum to the PAC from the PGVCB Clinical Working Group. January 17, 1996. Washington, D.C.

Blank AS, Gelsomino J. 1992. Persian Gulf veterans seen through VA's readjustment counseling service (RCS) vet centers and impact of the Persian Gulf War on VA's provision of readjustment counseling. Pp. 189–195 in Returning Persian Gulf Troops: First Year Findings. West Haven, Conn.: VA Northeast Program Evaluation Center.

Bolton HT. 1995. Use and safety of pesticides (repellents) in Persian Gulf. Presentation to the DVA: Update on health consequences of Persian Gulf service, Baltimore, Md., July 1995.

Brini CM, Tremblay GC. 1991. Reversible inhibition of the urea cycle and gluconeogenesis by *N,N*-diethyl-*m*-toluamide. Biochemical and Biophysical Research Communications 179:1264–1268.

Broadnax GB. 1992. Abortion rates post–Desert Storm. Memorandum to Colonel Ariel Rodriquez, Surgical Consultant, Office of the Surgeon General from Colonel Gary B. Broadnax. January 31, 1992. Washington, D.C.: Department of the Army, Office of the Surgeon General.

Caldwell GG. 1990. Twenty-two years of cancer cluster investigations at the Centers for Disease Control. American Journal of Epidemiology 132(Suppl 1):S43–S47.

Carmeli A, Liberman N, Mevorach L. 1991. Anxiety-related somatic reactions during missile attacks. Israel Journal of Medical Sciences 27:677–680.

Casida JE, Gammon DW, Glickman AH, Lawrence LJ. 1983. Mechanisms of selective action of pyrethroid insecticides. Annual Review of Pharmacology and Toxicology 23:413–438.

Coate BD, Anderson CM, Gray GC, Hyams KC, the Gulf War Veterans Research Team. 1995. Comparative study of hospitalizations among Gulf War veterans and era controls (abstract). Conference abstracts for 123rd annual meeting of the American Public Health Association, November 1995.

Cook JE, Kolka MA, Wenger CB. 1992. Chronic pyridostigmine bromide administration: Side effects among soldiers working in a dessert environment. Military Medicine 157:250–254.

Cowan DN, DeFraites R, Wishik S, Gray G, Kuhn J, the Gulf War Veterans Research Team. 1995. Birth defects and Persian Gulf War service: A preliminary analysis (abstract). Conference abstracts for 123rd annual meeting of the American Public Health Association, November 1995.

Crawford-Brown DJ, Wilson J. 1984. Observations on very long-term removal of uranium compounds. Health Physics 47:443–446.

Cullen MR. 1987. The worker with multiple chemical sensitivities: An overview. Occupational Medicine: State of the Art Reviews 2:655–661.

Cusick JJ. 1996. Request for information on possible use of leaded fuel in tent heaters during the Persian Gulf War. Memo to the Principal Deputy Assistant Secretary of Defense for Health Affairs, Department of Defense, from Lieutenant General Cusick. April 2, 1996. Washington, D.C.

Cutler JJ, Parker GS, Rosen S, Prenney B, Healey R, Caldwell GG. 1986. Childhood leukemia in Woburn, Massachusetts. Public Health Reports 101:201–205.

Daxon EG. 1993. Protocol for Monitoring Gulf War Veterans with Imbedded Fragments of Depleted Uranium. AFRRI Technical Report 93-2. Bethesda, Md.: Armed Forces Radiobiology Research Institute.

Daxon EG. 1994. DU Exposures during the Persian Gulf War. Presentation to NIH Technology Assessment Workshop Panel on the Persian Gulf Experience and Health. Bethesda, Md., April 1994.

Daxon EG, Musk JH. 1993. Assessment of the Risks from Imbedded Depleted Uranium Fragments. AFRRI Technical Report 93-1. Bethesda, Md.: Armed Forces Radiobiology Research Institute.

DeFraites RF, Wanat ER, Norwood AE, Williams S, Cowan D, Callahan T. 1992. Investigation of a Suspected Outbreak of an Unknown Disease Among Veterans of Operation Desert Shield/Storm, 123d Army Reserve Command, Fort Benjamin Harrison, Ind. Washington, D.C.: Walter Reed Army Institute of Research.

Derogatis LR, Melisaratos N. 1983. The brief symptom inventory: An introductory report. Psychological Medicine 13:595–605.

DHHS (Department of Health and Human Services). 1993. Dental amalgam: A scientific review and recommended Public Health Service strategy for research, education, and regulation. Final report of the Subcommittee on Risk Management of the Committee to Coordinate Environmental Health and Related Programs, Public Health Service, January 1993.

Diamond GL. 1989. Biological consequences of exposure to soluble forms of natural uranium. Radiation Protection Dosimetry 26:23–33.

DoD (Department of Defense). 1993. Health Consequences of the Exposure of Persian Gulf Force Members to the Fumes of Burning Oil. Report to the Congress.

DoD. 1995. Comprehensive Clinical Evaluation Program Report on 10,020 Participants. August 1995. Washington, D.C.: Department of Defense.

DoD. 1996. Comprehensive Clinical Evaluation Program for Persian Gulf War Veterans: CCEP Report on 18,598 Participants. April 2, 1996. Washington, D.C.: Department of Defense.

Donnay A. 1994. Correspondence to the Committee to Review the Health Consequences of Service During the Persian Gulf War, October 1994. IOM, Washington, D.C.

DSB (Defense Science Board). 1994. Final Report: Defense Science Board Task Force on Persian Gulf War Health Effects. Washington, D.C.: Office of the Under Secretary of Defense for Acquisition and Technology.

Dunn M. 1996. Governmental Investigations of Possible Exposure to Chemical and Biological Warfare Agents. Testimony to PAC, Atlanta, Ga., April 1996.

Dutton RE. 1995. Zoonotic diseases from the Persian Gulf War. Memorandum to the Commander, U.S. Army Medical Command, Fort Sam Houston, Tex. April 3, 1995.

DVA (Department of Veterans Affairs). 1995a. Minutes from meeting of the Persian Gulf Expert Scientific Panel. February 28, 1995.

DVA. 1995b. VA Manual. M-10, Part III, Chapters 1–4. Washington, DC.

Eells JT, Bandettini PA, Holman PA, Propp JM. 1992. Pyrethroid insecticide–induced alterations in mammalian synaptic membrane potential. Journal of Pharmacology and Experimental Therapeutics 262:1173–1181.

Eggert RW. 1994. Final Report of Robins AFB GA Investigation (TUA-T03704, 11–15 Apr 94). Memorandum from Major Russell W. Eggert. June 21, 1994. Department of the Air Force: Brooks Air Force Base, Tex.

Engel CC, Engel AL, Campbell SJ, McFall ME, Russo J, Katon W. 1993. Posttraumatic stress disorder symptoms and precombat sexual and physical abuse in Desert Storm veterans. Journal of Nervous and Mental Disease 181:683–688.

EPA (Environmental Protection Agency). 1991. Kuwait Oil Fires: Interagency Interim Report. Washington, D.C.: EPA.

Fishman AP. 1995. Correspondence to Office of Assistant Secretary of Defense, Health Affairs. April 6, 1995. Washington D.C.: Department of Defense.

Fletcher RH, Fletcher SW, Wagner EH. 1995. Clinical Epidemiology: The Essentials. 3rd ed. Baltimore: Williams and Wilkins.

Ford JD, Shaw D, Sennhauser S, Greaves D, Thacker B, Chandler P, McClain V, Schwartz L. 1992. Coming home for good: The Operation Desert Storm veterans and family psychosocial debriefing project. Pp. 153–176 in Returning Persian Gulf Troops: First Year Findings. West Haven, Conn.: VA Northeast Program Evaluation Center.

Fukuda K, Straus SE, Hickie I, Sharpe MC, Dobbins JG, Komaroff A, International Chronic Fatigue Syndrome Study Group. 1994. The chronic fatigue syndrome: A comprehensive approach to its definition and study. Annals of Internal Medicine 121:953–959.

GAO (U.S. General Accounting Office). 1993a. Operation Desert Storm. Army Not Adequately Prepared to Deal with Depleted Uranium Contamination. Washington, D.C.: GAO.

GAO. 1993b. Women in the Military: Deployment in the Persian Gulf War. Washington, D.C.: GAO.

Golding JM. 1994. Sexual assault history and physical health in randomly selected Los Angeles women. Health Psychology 13:130–138.

Goldstein G, Beers SR, Morrow LA, Shemansky WJ, Steinhauer SR. 1996. A preliminary neuropsychological study of Persian Gulf veterans. Journal of International Neuropsychological Society 2:368–371.

Gross MJ, Harrison JA. 1989. Some electrochemical features of the *in vivo* corrosion of dental amalgams. Journal of Applied Electrochemistry 19:301–310.

Haley R. 1995. Personal communication, October 1995.

Healy DL, Trounson AO, Andersen AN. 1994. Female infertility: Causes and treatment. Lancet 343:1539–1544.

Heick HMC, Peterson RG, Dalpe-Scott M, Qureshi IA. 1988. Insect repellent, *N,N*-diethyl-*m*-toluamide, effect on ammonia metabolism. Pediatrics 82:373–376.

Helmkamp JC. 1994. United States military casualty comparisons during the Persian Gulf War. Journal of Occupational Medicine 36:609–615.

Hines JF. 1993. A comparison of clinical diagnoses among male and female soldiers deployed during the Persian Gulf War. Military Medicine 158:99–101.

Holmes GP, Kaplan JE, Gantz NM, Komaroff AL, Schonberger LB, Straus SE, Jones JF, Dubois RE, Cunningham-Rundles C, Pahwa S, Tosato G, Zegans LS, Purtilo DT, Brown N, Schooley RT, Brus I. 1988. Chronic fatigue syndrome: A working case definition. Annals of Internal Medicine 108:387–389.

Horowitz MJ. 1986. Clinical Observations and Diagnoses. Pp. 13–42 in Stress Response Syndromes. 2nd ed. North Vale, N.J.: Jason Aronson.

Hyams KC, Hanson K, Wignall FS, Escamilla J, Oldfield EC. 1995. The impact of infectious diseases on the health of US troops deployed to the Persian Gulf during Operations Desert Shield and Desert Storm. Clinical Infectious Diseases 20:1497–1504.

Hyman ES. 1996. Presentation to PAC. San Antonio, Tex., February 27, 1996.

IOM (Institute of Medicine). 1995a. Committee to Review the Health Consequences of Service During the Persian Gulf War. Health Consequences of Service During the

Persian Gulf War: Initial Findings and Recommendations for Immediate Action. Washington, D.C.: National Academy Press.

IOM. 1995b. Committee on Defense Women's Health Research. Recommendations for Research on the Health of Military Women. Washington, D.C.: National Academy Press.

IOM. 1995c. Committee on Military Nutrition Research. Not Eating Enough: Overcoming Underconsumption of Military Operational Rations. Washington, D.C.: National Academy Press.

IOM. 1996. Committee on the DoD Persian Gulf Syndrome, Comprehensive Clinical Evaluation Program. Evaluation of the U.S. Department of Defense Persian Gulf Comprehensive Clinical Evaluation Program. Washington D.C.: National Academy Press.

Joseph S. 1996. Testimony to the Subcommittee on Human Resources and Intergovernmental Relations, Committee on Government Reform and Oversight, U.S. House of Representatives, June 25, 1996.

Kaiser KS, Hawksworth AW, Gray GC, the Gulf War Veterans Research Team. 1995. A comparison of self-reported symptoms among active duty Seabees: Gulf War veterans versus era controls (abstract). Conference abstracts for 123rd annual meeting of the American Public Health Association, November 1995.

Kang HK. 1996. PGHR information provided to IOM Committee to Review the Health Consequences of Service During the Persian Gulf War. IOM, Washington, D.C.

Kang HK, Bullman TA. 1995. A mortality follow-up study of Persian Gulf War veterans (abstract). Conference abstracts for 123rd annual meeting of the American Public Health Association, November 1995.

Kang HK, Dalager NA, Lee KY. 1995. PGHR information provided to IOM Committee to Review the Health Consequences of Service During the Persian Gulf War. IOM. Washington, D.C.

Keogh JP. 1995. DVA depleted uranium follow-up program—an update: Presentation to the VA Persian Gulf Expert Scientific Panel. Washington, D.C., June 27, 1995.

Kline J, Stein Z, Susser M. 1989. Conception to Birth. New York: Oxford University Press.

Kodavanti PRS, Mundy WR, Tilson HA, Harry GJ. 1993. Effects of selected neuroactive chemicals on calcium transporting systems in rat cerebellum and on survival of cerebellar granule cells. Fundamental and Applied Toxicology 21:308–316.

Koshes RJ, Rothberg, JM. 1994. Use of inpatient psychiatric services on a U.S. Army combat support post during Operations Desert Shield and Desert Storm: The stress of non-deployment. Military Medicine 159:454–456.

Kroenke K, Price RK. 1993. Symptoms in the community: Prevalence, classification, and psychiatric comorbidity. Archives of Internal Medicine 153:2474–2480.

Kuratsune H, Yamaguti K, Takahashi M, Misaki H, Tagawa S, Kitani T. 1994. Acylcarnitine deficiency in chronic fatigue syndrome. Clinical Infectious Diseases 18(Suppl 1):S62–S67.

Landry JR. 1996. Letter to Chairman of the Committee to Review the Health Consequences of Service in the Persian Gulf. From John R. Landry, National Intelligence Officer, General Purpose Forces, National Intelligence Council. Office of the Director of Central Intelligence, Washington, D.C. July 16, 1996.

Lasseter KC, Garg DC. 1996. A study to evaluate the safety, tolerance, pharmacokinetics and pharmacodynamics of pyridostigmine when given in single and multiple doses to males and females in different weight groups. Clinical/pharmacokinetic report prepared for USAMMDA, by Clinical Research Services and South Florida Drug Research Corporation.

Lavie P, Carmeli A, Mevorach L, Liberman N. 1991. Sleeping under the threat of the Scud: War-related environmental insomnia. Israeli Journal of Medical Science 27:681–686.

Lemasters GK, Pinney SM. 1989. Employment status as a confounder when assessing occupational exposures and spontaneous abortion. Journal of Clinical Epidemiology 42:975–981.

Lemieux AM, Coe CL. 1995. Abuse-related posttraumatic stress disorder: Evidence for chronic neuroendocrine activation in women. Psychosomatic Medicine 57:105–115.

Lillienfeld DE, Stolley PD. 1994. Foundations of Epidemiology. 3rd ed. New York: Oxford University Press.

Lloyd AR, Hickie I, Boughton CR, Spencer O, Wakefield D. 1990. Prevalence of chronic fatigue syndrome in an Australian population. Medical Journal of Australia 153:522–528.

Lotti M, Moretto A. 1995. Cholinergic symptoms and Gulf War syndrome (letter). Nature Medicine 1:1225–1226.

Magill AJ, Grögl M, Gasser RA, Sun W, Oster CN. 1993. Visceral infection caused by *Leishmania tropica* in veterans of Operation Desert Storm. New England Journal of Medicine 328:1383–1387.

Marlowe DH. 1996. Personal communication.

Marlowe DH. 1995. Stresses and the psychological consequences of Operation Desert Shield/Storm. Presentation to the IOM Committee to Review the Health Consequences of Service During the Persian Gulf War. Washington, D.C., June 1995.

Marlowe DH, Martin JA, Gifford RK. 1990a. Observations and Initial Findings of the WRAIR Stress Evaluation Team: Operation Desert Shield: September 22–October 6, 1990. Washington, D.C.: Department of Military Psychiatry, WRAIR.

Marlowe DH, Wright KM, Gifford RK, Belenky GL, Manning FJ, Leu J. 1990b. Second assessment: Soldier and unit adaptation, stress and human issues in Operation Desert Shield. Washington, D.C.: Department of Military Psychiatry, WRAIR.

Mather S. Testimony to PAC, May 1996. Washington, D.C.

Mattison DR. 1994. A framework for diagnosis: Reproductive and developmental toxicity. Presentation to NIH Technology Assessment Workshop Panel on the Persian Gulf Experience and Health, Bethesda, Md., April 1994.

McGill RG. 1993. Testimony to House VA Subcommittee on Oversight and Investigation on Health Issues and Gulf War Veterans. Washington, D.C., June 1993.

McGill RG. 1995. Memorandum dated January 31, 1995. Proposed multi-center multi-disciplinary collaboration to study "Gulf War Syndrome."

McGuire MC, Nogueira CP, Bartels CF, Lightstone H, Hajra A, et al. 1989. Identification of the structural mutation responsible for the dibucaine-resistant (atypical) variant form of human serum cholinesterase. Proceedings of the National Academy of Sciences 86:953–957.

Miller CS. 1994. Multiple chemical sensitivity and the Gulf War veterans. Presentation to NIH Technology Assessment Workshop Panel on the Persian Gulf Experience and Health, Bethesda, Md., April 1994.

Miller CS. 1996. Presentation to PAC. San Antonio, Tex.., February 1996.

Milner BI, Plezia RA. 1995. Toxic exposure sign: Desert Shield/Desert Storm. Cutis 55:289–290.

MMWR (Morbidity and Mortality Weekly Report). 1992. Viscerotropic leishmaniasis in persons returning from Operation Desert Storm—1990–1991. Morbidity and Mortality Weekly Report 41:131–134.

MMWR. 1995. Unexplained illness among Persian Gulf War veterans in an Air National Guard unit: Preliminary report—August 1990–March 1995. Morbidity and Mortality Weekly Report 44:443–448.

Moeller RB, Kalasinsky VF, Razzaque M, Centeno JA, Dick EJ, Abdal M, Petrov II, DeWitt TW, Al-Attar M, Pletcher JM, Briskey EJ. 1994. Assessment of the histopathological lesions and chemical analysis of feral cats to the smoke from the Kuwait oil fires. Journal of Environmental Pathology, Toxicology and Oncology 13:137–149.

Nathanson CA. 1975. Illness and the feminine role: A theoretical review. Social Science and Medicine 9:57–62.

Nathanson CA. 1980. Social roles and health status among women: the significance of employment. Social Science and Medicine 14A:463–471.

Nelson BJ, Hagedorn ME, Byron M. 1996. Rhythms of War: Activation experiences during the Persian Gulf War. Final Report to Tri-Service Nursing Program, Department of Defense, Washington, D.C.

NEPEC (Northeast Program Evaluation Center). 1992. Returning Persian Gulf Troops: First Year Findings. West Haven, Conn.: VA Northeast Program Evaluation Center.

Nicolson G. 1996. Presentation to PAC. San Antonio, Tex., February 1996.

Nicolson GL, Nicolson NL. 1995a. Doxycycline treatment and Desert Storm (letter). Journal of the American Medical Association 273:618–619.

Nicolson GL, Nicolson NL. 1995b. Mycoplasma infections in Gulf War illnesses. Presentation to PAC. Washington, D.C., August 1995.

NIH Technology Assessment Workshop Panel. 1994. The Persian Gulf experience and health. Journal of the American Medical Association 272:391–396.

NRC (National Research Council). 1983. Risk Assessment in the Federal Government: Managing the Process. Washington, D.C.: National Academy Press.

NRC. 1993. Issues in Risk Assessment. Washington, D.C.: National Academy Press.

O'Donnell FL. 1994. Environmental Conditions in Saudi Arabia. Presentation to NIH Technology Assessment Workshop Panel on the Persian Gulf Experience and Health, Bethesda, Md., April 1994.

Olshan AF, Faustman EM. 1993. Male-mediated developmental toxicity. Annual Review Public Health 14:159–181.

PAC (Presidential Advisory Committee). 1996a. Presidential Advisory Committee on Gulf War Veterans' Illnesses: Interim Report. Washington, D.C.: U.S. Government Printing Office.

PAC. 1996b. Transcript from meeting held April 16, 1996. Atlanta, Ga.

PAC. 1996c. Transcript from meeting held July 8–9, 1996. Chicago, Ill.

PAC. 1996d. Transcript from meeting held August 6, 1996. Denver, Colo.

Parkinson DK. 1992. Mercury. In: William N. Rom, ed., Environmental and Occupational Medicine. Boston: Little, Brown.

Penman AD, Tarver RS, Currier MM. 1996. No evidence of increase in birth defects and health problems among children born to Persian Gulf War veterans in Mississippi. Military Medicine 161:1–6.

Perconte ST, Wilson AT, Pontius EB, Dietrick AL, Spiro KJ. 1993. Psychological and war stress symptoms among deployed and non-deployed reservists following Persian Gulf War. Military Medicine 158:516–521.

Peterson R and Kalasinsky V. 1996. Personal communication.

PGVCB (Persian Gulf Veterans Coordinating Board). 1994. Summary of the Issues Impacting upon the Health of Persian Gulf Veterans, Version 3.0. Washington, D.C.: Support Office of the Persian Gulf Veterans Coordinating Board.

PGVCB. 1995a. Unexplained illnesses among Desert Storm Veterans. Archives of Internal Medicine 155:262–268.

PGVCB. 1995b. A Working Plan for Research on Persian Gulf Veterans' Illnesses. Washington, D.C., August, 1995.

PGVCB. 1995c. Persian Gulf Veterans Research Activity Report. Submitted by the Secretary of Veterans Affairs. Prepared for the Senate Veterans' Affairs Committee and the House Veterans' Affairs Committee, March 1995.

PGVCB RWG (Research Working Group). 1996. Annual Report to Congress. Federally sponsored research on Persian Gulf Veterans' Illnesses for 1995. Washington, D.C.

PGVIIT (Persian Gulf Veterans Illnesses Investigation Team). 1996. Coalition Chemical Detections and Health of Coalition Troops in Detection Area. Available on the Internet World Wide Web at http://www.dtic.dla.mil:80/gulflink/.

Pierce PF. 1995. Health and psychosocial readjustment of Gulf War veteran women. Scientific report of methods and selected preliminary findings.

Pierce PF. 1996. Physical and emotional health of Gulf War veteran women. Submitted for publication.

Pontius E, Wilson A, Perconte S, Spiro K, Dietrick A, et al. 1992. The need for continuing mental health intervention in soldiers returning from the Persian Gulf war: Assessment of deployed and non-deployed reserve units from western Pennsylvania, eastern Ohio, and West Virginia. Pp. 99–108 in Returning Persian Gulf Troops: First Year Findings. West Haven, Conn.: VA Northeast Program Evaluation Center.

Rappaport SM. 1993. Threshold limit values, permissible exposure limits, and feasibility: The bases for exposure limits in the United States. American Journal of Industrial Medicine 23:683–694.

Reeves W. Presentation to PAC. San Francisco, Calif., November 1995.

Richards AL, Hyams KC, Merrell BR, Dasch GA, Woody JN, Ksiazek TG, LeDuc JW, Watts DM. 1991. Medical aspects of Operation Desert Storm (letter). New England Journal of Medicine 325:970.

Richards AL, Malone JD, Sheris S, Weddle JR, Rossi CA, Ksiazek TG, LeDuc JW, Dasch GA, Hyams KC. 1993a. Arbovirus and rickettsial infections among combat troops during Operation Desert Shield/Desert Storm (letter). Journal of Infectious Diseases 168:1080–1081.

Richards AL, Hyams KC, Watts DM, Rozmajzl PJ, Woody JN, Merrell BR. 1993b. Respiratory disease among military personnel in Saudi Arabia during Operation Desert Shield. American Journal of Public Health 83:1326–1329.

Richardson RJ. 1995. Assessment of the neurotoxic potential of chlorpyrifos relative to other organophosphorus compounds: A critical review of the literature. Journal of Toxicology and Environmental Health 44:135–165.

Riley EB. 1992. Operation Desert Shield/Desert Storm. History of Participation by the U.S. Army Environmental Hygiene Agency, Aberdeen Proving Ground, Maryland (August 7, 1990–December 31, 1991). Aberdeen Proving Ground, Md.: USAEHA.

Robbins PJ, Cherniack MG. 1986. Review of the biodistribution and toxicity of the insect repellent *N,N*-diethyl-*m*-toluamide (DEET). Journal of Toxicology and Environmental Health 18:503–525.

Rodell DE, Cooley KD, West LT, Altheimer EL. 1992. The Persian Gulf outreach program at the Little Rock VA Medical Center. Pp. 77–98 in Returning Persian Gulf Troops: First Year Findings. West Haven, Conn.: VA Northeast Program Evaluation Center.

Rosa C. 1993. Spontaneous abortion rate and the Gulf War mobilization. Journal U.S. Army Medical Department Sept/Oct.:6–7, 14.

Rothman KJ. 1990. A sobering start for the cluster busters' conference. American Journal of Epidemiology 132(Suppl 1):S6–S13.

Rowe PC, Bou-Holaigah I, Kan JS, Calkins H. 1995. Is neurally mediated hypotension an unrecognized cause of chronic fatigue? Lancet 345:623–624.

Savitz DA, Whelan EA, Rowland AS, Kleckner RC. 1990. Maternal employment and reproductive risk factors. American Journal of Epidemiology 132:933–45.

Schrader SM, Kesner JS. 1993. Male reproductive toxicology. In Paul M ed., Occupational and Environmental Reproductive Hazards: A Guide for Clinicians. Baltimore, Md. Williams & Wilkins.

Schull WJ. 1996. Psychosocial concerns. In William J. Schull, ed., Effects of Atomic Radiation: A Half-Century of Studies from Hiroshima and Nagasaki. New York: Wiley-Liss.

Scialli AR. 1992. A Clinical Guide to Reproductive and Developmental Toxicology. Boca Raton, Fla.: CRC Press.

Scotti JR, Beach BK, Northrop LME, Forsyth JP, Rode CA, Szymanski LA, Beeler LL, Cornell KM, Price K, Thompson J. 1993. An investigation of the effects of involvement in Operation Desert Storm: Psychological distress in the veteran, spouse, and children. Presented at the annual convention of the Association for the Advancement of Behavior Therapy, November 1993. Atlanta, Ga.

Selye H. 1956. The Stress of Life. New York: McGraw-Hill.

Sharpe MC, Archard LC, Banatvala JE, Borysiewicz LK, Clare AW, David A, Edwards RHT, Hawton KEH, Lambert HP, Lane RJM, McDonald EM, Mowbray JF, Pearson DJ, Peto TEA, Preedy VR, Smith AP, Smith DG, Taylor DJ, Tyrrell DAJ, Wessely S, White PD. 1991. A report—chronic fatigue syndrome: Guidelines for research. Journal of the Royal Society of Medicine 84:118–121.

Shepard TH, Fantel AG, Mirkes PE. 1993. Developmental toxicology: Prenatal period. In M Paul, ed., Occupational and Environmental Reproductive Hazards: A Guide for Clinicians. Baltimore, Md. Williams & Wilkins.

Skakkebaek NE, Giwercman A, de Kretser D. 1994. Pathogenesis and management of male infertility. Lancet 343:1473–1479.

Sloan P, Arsenault L, McCormick WA, Dunn S, Scalf L. 1992. Initial contact interviews with Marine reservists in Operation Desert Storm. Pp. 143–151 in Returning Persian Gulf Troops: First Year Findings. West Haven, Conn.: VA Northeast Program Evaluation Center.

Sloan P, Arsenault L, Hilsenroth M, Harvill L. 1995a. Use of Mississippi Scale for combat-related PTSD in detecting war-related, non-combat stress symptomatology. Journal of Clinical Psychology 51:799–801.

Sloan P, Arsenault L, Hilsenroth M, Harvill L, Handler L. 1995b. Rorschach measures of posttraumatic stress in Persian Gulf War veterans. Journal of Personality Assessment 64:397–414.

Sloan P, Arsenault L, Hilsenroth M, Harvill L. 1996a. Assessment of noncombat, war-related posttraumatic stress symptomatology: Validity of the PK, PS, and IES scales. Psychological Assessment 3:37–41.

Sloan P, Arsenault L, Hilsenroth M, Harvill L. 1996b. Rorschach measures of posttraumatic stress in Persian Gulf war veterans: A three year follow-up study. Journal of Personality Assessment 66:54–64.

Sohler P, Smith L, Welk R, Stacey R, Godown I. 1992. Psychological adjustment in ODS/S veterans. Pp. 177–188 in Returning Persian Gulf Troops: First Year Findings. West Haven, Conn.: VA Northeast Program Evaluation Center.

Sorensen KA, Feild TC. 1994. Projections of the U.S. veteran population: 1990 to 2010. Statistical Brief. Washington, D.C.: Department of Veterans Affairs.

Southwick S, Morgan A. 1992. West Haven VA Medical Center Operation Desert Storm report. Pp. 69–76 in Returning Persian Gulf Troops: First Year Findings. West Haven, Conn.: VA Northeast Program Evaluation Center.

Southwick SM, Morgan A, Nagy LM, Bremner D, Nicolaou AL, Johnson DR, Rosenheck R, Charney DS. 1993. Trauma-related symptoms in veterans of Operation Desert Storm: A preliminary report. American Journal of Psychiatry 150:1524–1528.

Sparks PJ, Daniell W, Black DW, Kipen HM, Altman LC, Simon GE, Terr AI. 1994. Multiple chemical sensitivity syndrome: A clinical perspective. I. Case definition, theories of pathogenesis, and research needs. Journal Occupational Medicine 36:718–730.

Stevens CG. 1995. Zoonotic diseases from the Persian Gulf War. Memorandum to the Assistant Secretary of Defense (Health Affairs) from Colonel Charles G. Stevens, Department of the Army Office of the Surgeon General. April 25, 1995.

Straus SE. 1991. History of chronic fatigue syndrome. Review of Infectious Diseases 13(Suppl 1):S2–S7.

Stretch RH, Bliese PD, Marlowe DH, Wright KM, Knudson KH, Hoover CH. 1995. Physical health symptomatology of Gulf War-era service personnel from the states of Pennsylvania and Hawaii. Military Medicine 160:131–136.

Stretch RH, Bliese PD, Marlowe DH, Wright KM, Knudson KH, Hoover CH. 1996. Psychological health of Gulf War-era military personnel. Military Medicine 161:257–261.

Summers AO. 1994. Letter to Dr. John Bailar dated April 17, 1994.

Summers AO, Wireman J, Vimy MJ, Lorscheider FL, Marshall B, Levy SB, Bennett S, Billard L. 1993. Mercury released from dental "silver" fillings provokes an increase in mercury- and antibiotic-resistant bacteria in oral and intestinal floras of primates. Antimicrobial Agents and Chemotherapy 37:825–834.

Sutker PB, Uddo M, Brailey K, Allain AN. 1992. Operation Desert Shield/Storm (ODS) Returnee Evaluation, Debriefing, and Treatment Program Report. Pp. 45–68 in Returning Persian Gulf Troops: First Year Findings. West Haven, Conn.: VA Northeast Program Evaluation Center.

Sutker PB, Uddo M, Brailey K, Allain AN. 1993. War-zone trauma and stress-related symptoms in Operation Desert Shield/Storm (ODS) returnees. Journal of Social Issues 49:33–49.

Sutker PB, Uddo M, Brailey K, Allain AN, Errera P. 1994a. Psychological symptoms and psychiatric diagnoses in Operation Desert Storm troops serving graves registration duty. Journal of Traumatic Stress 7:159–171.

Sutker PB, Uddo M, Brailey K, Vasterling JJ, Errera P. 1994b. Psychopathology in war-zone deployed and nondeployed Operation Desert Storm troops assigned graves registration duties. Journal of Abnormal Psychology 103:383–390.

Sutker PB, Davis JM, Uddo M, Ditta SR. 1995a. Assessment of psychological distress in Persian Gulf troops: Ethnicity and gender comparisons. Journal of Personality Assessment 64:415–427.

Sutker PB, Uddo M, Davis JM, Ditta SR. 1995b. War zone stress, personal resources, and PTSD in Persian Gulf War returnees. Journal of Abnormal Psychology 104:444–452.

Tuite J. 1996. Testimony to the Presidential Advisory Committee on Gulf War Veterans' Illnesses, April 1996. Atlanta, Ga.

U.S. Congress Office of Technology Assessment. 1993. The Department of Veterans Affairs PG Veterans' Health Registry, OTA-H-577, Washington, D.C.

U.S. Congress Office of Technology Assessment. 1994. The Department of Defense Kuwait Oil Fire Health Risk Assessment, BP-H-138, Washington, D.C.

U.S. Gulf Environmental Technical Assistance. 1992. Report to Congress.

UN (United Nations). 1995. Report of the Secretary General on the Status of the Implementation of the Special Commission's Plan for the Ongoing Monitoring and Verification of Iraq's Compliance with Relevant Parts of Section C of Security Council Resolution 687 (1991). New York: United Nations.

Unger WS, Shea MT, Curran JP. 1992. An evaluation of troops returning from the Persian Gulf: A preliminary report. Pp. 131–142 in Returning Persian Gulf Troops: First Year Findings. West Haven, Conn.: VA Northeast Program Evaluation Center.

USACHPPM (U.S. Army Center for Health Promotion and Preventive Medicine). 1995. Acute Oral Toxicity Study of Pyridostigmine Bromide, Permethrin, and DEET in the Laboratory Rat. Toxicological study 75-48-2665. Washington, D.C., May 31, 1995.

USAEHA (U.S. Army Environmental Hygiene Agency). 1992. Interim Kuwait Oil Fire Health Risk Assessment, No. 39-26-L192-91, May 5–September 15, 1991. Aberdeen Proving Ground, Md.:USAEHA.

USAEHA. 1994. Final Report—Kuwait Oil Fire Health Risk Assessment, No. 39-26-L192-91, 5 May–3 December 1991. Aberdeen Proving Ground, Md.: USAEHA.

USAMRMC (U.S. Army Medical Research and Materiel Command). 1994. The General Well-Being of Gulf War Era Service Personnel from the States of Pennsylvania and Hawaii: A Survey. Washington, D.C.: Walter Reed Army Institute of Research.

VA (Veterans Administration). 1985. Survey of Female Veterans: A Study of the Needs, Attitudes, and Experiences of Women Veterans. Washington, D.C.: Veterans Administration.

Vijverberg HPM, van den Bercken J. 1990. Neurotoxicological effects and the mode of action of pyrethroid insecticides. Critical Reviews in Toxicology 21:105–126.

Vogt T, Pope C, Mullooly J, Hollis J. 1994. Mental health status as a predictor of morbidity and mortality: A 15-year follow-up of members of a health maintenance organization. American Journal of Public Health 84(2):227–231.

WMO (World Meteorological Organization). 1991. Report of the WMO meeting of experts on the atmospheric part of the joint UN response to the Kuwait oilfield fires. Geneva, Switzerland, April 1991.

WMO. 1992. Report of the second WMO meeting of experts to assess the response to and atmospheric effects of the Kuwait oil fires. Geneva, Switzerland, May 1992.

Wolfe F, Smythe HA, Yunus MB, Bennett RM, Bombardier C, et al. 1990. The American College of Rheumatogy 1990 criteria for the classification of fibromyalgia: Report of the Multicenter Criteria Committee. Arthritis and Rheumatism 33:160–172.

Wolfe J, Brown PJ, Bucsela ML. 1992a. Symptom responses of female Vietnam veterans to Operation Desert Storm. American Journal of Psychiatry 149:676–679.

Wolfe J, Young BL, Brown PJ. 1992b. Self-reported sexual assault in female Gulf War veterans. Presented at the 123rd annual meeting of the Association for the Advancement of Behavior Therapy, November 1992.

Wolfe J, Kelley JM, Bucsela ML, Mark WR. 1992c. Fort Devens Reunion Survey: report of phase I. Pp. 19–44 in Returning Persian Gulf Troops: First Year Findings. West Haven, Conn.: VA Northeast Program Evaluation Center.

Wolfe J, Brown PJ, Kelley JM. 1993. Reassessing war stress: Exposure and the Persian Gulf War. Journal of Social Issues 49:15–31.

Wolfe J, Proctor SP, Brown P, Kimerling R, Duncan J, Sullivan M, Chrestman K, White RF. 1994. Relationship of physical health and post-traumatic stress disorder in young adult women. Poster presented at the Annual Meeting of the American Psychological Association's Conference on Psychosocial and Behavioral Factors in Women's Health, May 1994.

Wolfe J, Proctor S, Sullivan M, Duncan-Davis J. 1995. Posttraumatic stress and physical health: Does gender play a role? Poster presentation, Harvard Medical School.

WRAIR (Walter Reed Army Institute of Research). 1992. Human factors research in Desert Shield/Storm. Briefing prepared for DIV CDR 101st ABN DIV (AA), Fort Campbell, Ky. Washington, D.C.: Department of Psychiatry, WRAIR.

Wright KM, Marlowe DH, Gifford RK. 1991. Operation Desert Shield Preparation for the War: Deployment Stresses. Washington, D.C.: Department of Military Psychiatry, WRAIR.

Writer JV, DeFraites RF, Brundage JF. 1996. Comparative mortality among US military personnel in the Persian Gulf region and worldwide during Operations Desert Shield and Desert Storm. Journal of the American Medical Association 275:118–121.

Wynd CA, Dziedzicki RE. 1992. Heightened anxiety in army reserve nurses anticipating mobilization during Operation Desert Storm. Military Medicine 157:630–634.

Wyngaarden JB, Smith LH, Bennett JC, eds. 1992. Cecil Textbook of Medicine, Vol. 2. 19th ed. Philadelphia: W. B. Saunders.

Yehuda R, Giller EL, Mason JW. 1993. Psychoneuroendocrine assessment of posttraumatic stress disorder: Current progress and new directions. Progress in Neuro-Psychopharmacology and Biological Psychiatry 17:541–550.

Young RC, Rachal RE, Huguley JW. 1992. Environmental health concerns of the Persian Gulf War. Journal of the National Medical Association 84:417–424.

Ziem GE. 1992. Multiple chemical sensitivity: Treatment and follow-up with avoidance and control of chemical exposures. Toxicology and Industrial Health 8:73–86.

Ziem GE. 1994. Public meeting presentation to the Committee to Review the Health Consequences of Service During the Persian Gulf War, February 1994. IOM, Washington, D.C.

Appendixes

A

Relevant Sections of Public Law 102-585

PL 102-585 PERSIAN GULF WAR VETERANS' HEALTH STATUS

SEC. 702. PERSIAN GULF WAR VETERANS HEALTH REGISTRY.

(a) ESTABLISHMENT OF REGISTRY.—The Secretary of Veterans Affairs shall establish and maintain a special record to be known as the "Persian Gulf War Veterans Health Registry" (in this section referred to as the "Registry").

(b) CONTENTS OF REGISTRY.—Except as provided in subsection (c), the Registry shall include the following information:

(1) A list containing the name of each individual who served as a member of the Armed Forces in the Persian Gulf theater of operations during the Persian Gulf War and who—

(A) applies for care or services from the Department of Veterans Affairs under chapter 17 of title 38, United States Code;

(B) files a claim for compensation under chapter 11 of such title on the basis of any disability which may be associated with such service;

(C) dies and is survived by a spouse, child, or parent who files a claim for dependency and indemnity compensation under chapter 13 of such title on the basis of such service;

(D) requests from the Department a health examination under section 703; or

(E) receives from the Department of Defense a health examination similar to the health examination referred to in subparagraph (D) and requests inclusion in the Registry.

(2) Relevant medical data relating to the health status of, and other information that the Secretary considers relevant and appropriate with respect to, each individual described in paragraph (1) who—

(A) grants to the Secretary permission to include such information in the Registry; or

(B) at the time the individual is listed in the Registry, is deceased.

(c) INDIVIDUALS SUBMITTING CLAIMS OR MAKING REQUESTS BEFORE DATE OF ENACTMENT.—If in the case of an individual described in subsection (b)(1) the application, claim, or request referred to in such subsection was submitted, filed, or made, before the date of the enactment of this Act, the Secretary shall, to the extent feasible, include in the Registry such individual's name and the data and information, if any, described in subsection (b)(2) relating to the individual.

(d) DEPARTMENT OF DEFENSE INFORMATION.—The Secretary of Defense shall furnish to the Secretary of Veterans Affairs such information maintained by the Department of Defense as the Secretary of Veterans Affairs considers necessary to establish and maintain the Registry.

(e) RELATION TO DEPARTMENT OF DEFENSE REGISTRY.—The Secretary of Veterans Affairs, in consultation with the Secretary of Defense, shall ensure that information is collected and maintained in the Registry in a manner that permits effective and efficient cross-reference between the Registry and the registry established under section 734 of the National Defense Authorization Act for Fiscal Years 1992 and 1993 (Public Law 102-190; 105 Stat. 1411; 10 U.S.C. 1074 note), as amended by section 704.

(f) ONGOING OUTREACH TO INDIVIDUALS LISTED IN REGISTRY.—The Secretary of Veterans Affairs shall, from time to time, notify individuals listed in the Registry of significant developments in research on the health consequences of military service in the Persian Gulf theater of operations during the Persian Gulf War.

SEC. 703. HEALTH EXAMINATIONS AND COUNSELING FOR VETERANS ELIGIBLE FOR INCLUSION IN CERTAIN HEALTH-RELATED REGISTRIES.

(a) In General.—(1) The Secretary of Veterans Affairs—

(A) shall, upon the request of a veteran described in subsection (b)(1), provide the veteran with a health examination and consultation and counseling with respect to the results of the examination; and

(B) may, upon the request of a veteran described in subsection (b)(2), provide the veteran with such an examination and such consultation and counseling.

(2) The Secretary shall carry out appropriate outreach activities with respect to the provision of any health examinations and consultations and counseling services under paragraph (1).

(b) COVERED VETERANS.—(1) In accordance with subsection (a)(1)(A), the Secretary shall provide an examination, consultation, and counseling under that subsection to any veteran who is eligible for listing or inclusion in the Persian Gulf War Veterans Health Registry established by section 702.

(2) In accordance with subsection (a)(1)(B), the Secretary may provide an examination, consultation, and counseling under that subsection to any veteran who is eligible for listing or inclusion in any other similar health-related registry administered by the Secretary.

SEC. 704. EXPANSION OF COVERAGE OF PERSIAN GULF REGISTRY.

(a) IN GENERAL.—Subsections (a) and (b) of section 734 of the National Defense Authorization Act for Fiscal Years 1992 and 1993 (Public Law 102-190; 105 Stat. 1411; 10 U.S.C. 1074 note) are amended to read as follows:

"(a) ESTABLISHMENT OF REGISTRY.—The Secretary of Defense shall establish and maintain a special record (in this section referred to as the 'Registry') relating to the following members of the Armed Forces:

"(1) Members who, as determined by the Secretary, were exposed to the fumes of burning oil in the Operation Desert Storm theater of operations during the Persian Gulf conflict.

"(2) Any other members who served in the Operation Desert Storm theater of operations during the Persian Gulf conflict.

"(b) CONTENTS OF REGISTRY.—(1) The Registry shall include—

"(A) with respect to each class of members referred to in each of paragraphs (1) and (2) of subsection (a) —

"(i) a list containing each such member's name and other relevant identifying information with respect to the member; and

"(ii) to the extent that data are available and inclusion of the data is feasible, a description of the circumstances of the member's service during the Persian Gulf conflict, including the locations in the Operation Desert Storm theater of operations in which such service occurred and the atmospheric and other environmental circumstances in such locations at the time of such service; and

"(B) with respect to the members referred to in subsection (a)(1), a description of the circumstances of each exposure of each such member to the fumes of burning oil as described in such subsection (a)(1), including the length of time of the exposure.

"(2) The Secretary shall establish the Registry with the advice of an independent scientific organization."

(b) CONFORMING AMENDMENTS.—(1) Subsection (c)(1) of such section is amended by striking out "subsection (a)" and inserting in lieu thereof "subsection (a)(1)."

(2) Subsection (d) of such section is amended by inserting "pursuant to subsection (a)(1)" after "Registry."

SEC. 706. AGREEMENT WITH NATIONAL ACADEMY OF SCIENCES FOR REVIEW OF HEALTH CONSEQUENCES OF SERVICE DURING THE PERSIAN GULF WAR.

(a) AGREEMENT.—(1) The Secretary of Veterans Affairs and Secretary of Defense jointly shall seek to enter into an agreement with the National Academy of Sciences for the Medical Follow-Up Agency (MFUA) of the Institute of Medicine of the Academy to review existing scientific, medical, and other information on the health consequences of military service in the Persian Gulf theater of operations during the Persian Gulf War.

(2) The agreement shall require MFUA to provide members of veterans organizations and members of the scientific community (including the Director of the Office of Technology Assessment) with the opportunity to comment on the method or methods MFUA proposes to use in conducting the review.

(3) The agreement shall permit MFUA, in conducting the review, to examine and evaluate medical records of individuals who are included in the registries referred to in section 705(d) for purposes that MFUA considers appropriate, including the purpose of identifying illnesses of those individuals.

(4) The Secretary of Veterans Affairs and the Secretary of Defense shall seek to enter into the agreement under this section not later than 180 days after the date of the enactment of this Act.

(b) REPORT.—(1) The agreement under this section shall require the National Academy of Sciences to submit to the committees and secretaries referred to in paragraph (2) a report on the results of the review carried out under the agreement. Such report shall contain the following:

(A) An assessment of the effectiveness of actions taken by the Secretary of Veterans Affairs and the Secretary of Defense to collect and maintain information that is potentially useful for assessing the health consequences of the military service referred to in subsection (a).

(B) Recommendations on means of improving the collection and maintenance of such information.

(C) Recommendations on whether there is sound scientific basis for an epidemiological study or studies on the health consequences of such service, and if the recommendation is that there is sound scientific basis for such a study or studies, the nature of the study or studies.

(2) The committees and secretaries referred to in paragraph (1) are the following:

(A) The Committees on Veterans' Affairs of the Senate and House of Representatives.

(B) The Committees on Armed Services of the Senate and House of Representatives.

(C) The Secretary of Veterans Affairs.

(D) The Secretary of Defense.

(c) FUNDING.—(1) The Secretary of Veterans Affairs and the Secretary of Defense shall make available up to a total of $500,000 in fiscal year 1993, from funds available to the Department of Veterans Affairs and the Department of Defense in that fiscal year, to carry out the review. Any amounts provided by the two departments shall be provided in equal amounts.

(2) If the Secretary of Veterans Affairs and the Secretary of Defense enter into an agreement under subsection (a) with the National Academy of Sciences—

(A) the Secretary of Veterans Affairs shall make available $250,000 in each of fiscal years 1994 through 2003, from amounts available to the Department of Veterans Affairs in each such fiscal year, to the National Academy of Sciences for the general purposes of conducting epidemiological research with respect to military and veterans populations; and

(B) the Secretary of Defense shall make available $250,000 in each of fiscal years 1994 through 2003, from amounts available to the Department of Defense in each such fiscal year, to the National Academy of Sciences for the purposes of carrying out the research referred to in subparagraph (A).

SEC. 707. COORDINATION OF GOVERNMENT ACTIVITIES ON HEALTH-RELATED RESEARCH ON THE PERSIAN GULF WAR.

(a) DESIGNATION OF COORDINATING ORGANIZATION.—The President shall designate, and may redesignate from time to time, the head of an appropriate department or agency of the Federal Government to coordinate all research activities undertaken or funded by the Executive Branch of the Federal Government on the health consequences of military service in the Persian Gulf theater of operations during the Persian Gulf War.

(b) REPORT.—Not later than March 1 of each year, the head of the department or agency designated under subsection (a) shall submit to the Committees on Veterans' Affairs of the Senate and House of Representatives a report on the status and results of all such research activities undertaken or by the Executive Branch of the Federal Government during the previous year.

B

Statement of Task

As directed by Public Law 102-585, passed by Congress in November 1992, the Institute of Medicine of the National Academy of Sciences will form a committee to review "existing scientific, medical and other information on the health consequences of military service in the Persian Gulf theater of operations during the Persian Gulf War." The Committee to Review the Health Consequences of Service During the Persian Gulf War has been charged to:

- assess the effectiveness of actions taken by the Secretary of Veterans Affairs and Secretary of Defense to collect and maintain information that is potentially useful for assessing the health consequences of the military service referred to in subsection (a) of P.L. 102-585;
- make recommendations on means of improving the collection and maintenance of such information; and
- make recommendations as to whether there is sound scientific basis for an epidemiological study or studies on the health consequences of such service, and if the recommendation is that there is sound scientific basis for such a study or studies, the nature of the study or studies.

In order to be informed from multiple sources, the committee will review relevant scientific literature and other information and will hold public meetings and scientific workshops. The committee will conduct a three year study and prepare a final report.

SPONSORS: Department of Veterans Affairs and Department of Defense

November 5, 1993
(date of statement) (date of previous statement, if applicable)

C

Committee Meetings and Individuals Providing Information

Committee meeting dates and locations

January 20–21, 1994, Washington, D.C.
February 28–March 1, 1994, Washington, D.C. (public meeting)
April 20–21, 1994, Washington, D.C.
July 14–16, 1994, Irvine, Calif.
August 30–September 1, 1994, Washington, D.C.
January 25–26, 1995, Washington, D.C.
March 9, 1995, Washington, D.C.
May 3–4, 1995, Washington, D.C.
June 19–20, 1995, Washington, D.C.
September 27–29, 1995, Woods Hole, Mass.
January 31–February 2, 1996, Irvine, Calif.
March 27–28, 1996, Washington, D.C.
April 24, 1996, Washington, D.C.
May 20–21, 1996, Woods Hole, Mass.

Presenters at the public meeting

Mrs. Kelli Albuck, spouse of Troy Albuck, Barrington, Ill.
Mr. Troy Albuck, Persian Gulf (PG) veteran, Barrington, Ill.
Ms. Helen Ellis, mother of PG veteran, Oakton, Va.
Mr. Paul Guerrette, PG veteran, Petersburg, Va.
Mr. Richard Haines, Army Reservist, New Albany, Ind.

Mr. Kimo Hollingsworth, PG veteran, American Legion, Washington, D.C.
Ms. Mary Lamielle, National Center for Environmental Health Strategies, Vorhees, N.J.
Ms. Penny Larrisey, spouse of PG veteran, Philadelphia, Pa.
Mr. Steve Robertson, PG veteran, American Legion, Washington, D.C.
Dr. Herbert Smith, PG veteran, Ijamsville, Md.
Dr. Grace Ziem, occupational medicine physician, Baltimore, Md.

Sources of written testimony for the public meeting

Ms. Venus-Valiery Hammack, PG veteran, Lowell, Mass.
Ms. Evelyn Hazen, U.S. Army (retired), Walla Walla, Wash.
Mr. Tad Leeds, PG veteran, Decatur, Ga.
Ms. Jeanette Martinez, Operation Desert Shield/Storm Association, and widow of PG veteran, San Antonio, Tex.
Dr. Ruth Gordon McGill, San Angelo, Tex.
Ms. Janelle Payne, spouse of PG veteran, Glendale, Ariz.
Mr. Anthony Picou, Jr., Operation Desert Shield/Storm Association, San Antonio, Tex.
Mr. Nick Roberts, PG veteran, Phoenix City, Ariz.
Mr. Paul Sullivan, PG veteran, Atlanta, Ga.
MAJ Chris Wilman, U.K. Ministry of Defense, British Embassy, Washington, D.C.

Sources of other materials

Mrs. Gwen Allen, PG veteran, Mt. Vernon, Ind.
Dr. Rupert Ammann, Fort Collins, Colo.
Ms. Dorothy L. Brooks, Buies Creek, N.C.
Dr. Andrew M. Brown, Gadsden, Ala.
Mr. Len Dart, Nashua, N.H.
Mr. Albert Donnay, Baltimore, Md.
Dr. John Ellis, family member of PG veteran, Oakton, Va.
Mr. Joseph Ellis, PG veteran, Gainesville, Fla.
Ms. Francis Juanice Fox, family member of PG veteran, Phoenix, Ariz.
Dr. Kendall Gerdes, Denver, Colo.
LTC John T. Graham, director of Defense Medicine Services, U.K.
Mr. Michael Gray, Houston, Tex.
Mrs. Vickie Gray, Houston, Tex.
Mr. David Greenleaf, Island Pond, Vt.
Ms. Joan Marie Grimes, PG veteran, Washington, D.C.
Ms. Evelyn Hazen, PG veteran, Walla Walla, Wash.
Mr. Solomon Jamerson, U.S. Army (retired), Los Angeles, Calif.
Dr. Alexander Karczmar, Hines, Ill.

Dr. Sanford F. Kuvin, Palm Beach, Fla.
Mr. Martin Lee, Jr., Patlow, Va.
Mr. Tad Leeds, PG veteran, Decatur, Ga.
Dr. Ruth McGill, San Angelo, Tex.
Ms. Betty Mekdeci, Orlando, Fla.
Dr. Arthur Mende, Vadnais Heights, Minn.
Mr. Don Mills, Portland, Oreg.
Dr. Boaz Milner, Allen Park, Mich.
Dr. Joseph Neumann, Mountain Home, Tenn.
Dr. Patricia Olson, staff to Senate Veterans Affairs Committee, Washington, D.C.
Mr. T.M. Roche, U.K.
Ms. Mary Shears, spouse of PG veteran, Cedar Rapids, Iowa
Dr. Donald Stewart, Alfred, N.Y.
Dr. Anne Summers, Athens, Ga.
Dr. Andrew Urbanc, Fallbrook, Calif.
Mr. Lenny Woodard, PG veteran, Texarkana, Ark.

D

Invited Presentations

Dr. Miriam Alter, Centers for Disease Control and Prevention, Atlanta, Ga.
Mr. Fred Ambrose, Defense Intelligence Agency, Washington, D.C.
Dr. Maria Araneta, Naval Health Research Center, San Diego, Calif.
Dr. Drue Barrett, Centers for Disease Control and Prevention, Atlanta, Ga.
Dr. Arthur Barsky, Brigham and Women's Hospital, Harvard Medical School, Boston, Mass.
Dr. William Baumzweiger, Encino, Calif.
CAPT William Berg, MC, Navy Environmental and Preventive Medicine Unit No 2, Norfolk, Va.
MAJ Stephen Berté, U.S. Army Medical Materiel Development Activity, Fort Detrick, Md.
Dr. Sal Bosco, Defense Science Board Task Force on Chemical Weapons, Washington, D.C.
Dr. Dennis Bourdette, Department of Veterans Affairs (DVA) Environmental Health Research Center, Portland, Oreg.
Dr. Kelly Brix, Institute of Medicine, Washington, D.C.
COL John Brundage, MC, U.S. Army Center for Health Promotion and Preventive Medicine, Aberdeen Proving Ground, Md.
Ms. Rebecca Calderon, Naval Health Research Center, San Diego, Calif.
Dr. David Cowan, Walter Reed Army Institute of Research, Washington, D.C.
COL Frank Cox, Defense Science Board Task Force on Chemical Weapons, Washington, D.C.

LTC Robert DeFraites, MC, Walter Reed Army Institute of Research, Washington, D.C.

Dr. Larry Dlugosz, Naval Health Research Center, San Diego, Calif.

Mr. Layne Drash, DVA Central Office, Washington, D.C.

LTC Edward Eitzen, MC, U.S. Army Medical Research Institute of Infectious Diseases, Frederick, Md.

Lt Col Gary Gackstetter, Department of Defense, Office of the Assistant Secretary of Defense, Health Affairs, Washington, D.C.

Dr. Frank Garland, Naval Health Research Center, San Diego, Calif.

Dr. Timothy Gerrity, DVA Central Office, Washington, D.C.

CDR Gregory C. Gray, MC, Naval Health Research Center, San Diego, Calif.

Mr. Don Hakenson, U.S. Army Joint Services Environmental Support Group, Ft. Belvoir, Va.

Dr. Jack Heller, U.S. Army Center for Health Promotion and Preventive Medicine, Aberdeen Proving Ground, Md.

Dr. Rogene Henderson, National Academy of Sciences, Committee on Toxicology, Washington, D.C.

LTC Carl Hendricks, Director, Patient Administration Systems and Biostatistical Activity, Ft. Sam Houston, Tex.

Ms. Kathy Hiliopoulos, Naval Health Research Center, San Diego, Calif.

COL Charles G. Hurst, MC, Medical Research Institute of Chemical Defense, Aberdeen Proving Ground, Md.

Mr. Kevin Kaiser, Naval Health Research Center, San Diego, Calif.

Dr. Han Kang, DVA Central Office, Washington, D.C.

Ms. Deborah Katz, Institute of Medicine, Washington, D.C.

Dr. Howard Kipen, Robert Wood Johnson Medical School, Piscataway, N.J.

Dr. Kurt Kroenke, Uniformed Services University of Health Sciences, Bethesda, Md.

MAJ William Legg, U.S. Army Environmental Hygiene Agency, Aberdeen Proving Ground, Md.

Dr. Stanley Lemon, University of North Carolina, Chapel Hill

LTC Alan Magill, MC, Walter Reed Army Institute of Research, Washington, D.C.

Dr. David Marlowe, Walter Reed Army Institute of Research, Washington, D.C.

Dr. Boaz Milner, VA Medical Center, Allen Park, Mich.

Dr. Frances Murphy, DVA Central Office, Washington, D.C.

Dr. Benjamin Natelson, DVA Environmental Health Research Center, East Orange, N.J.

Dr. Neil Otchin, DVA Central Office, Washington, D.C.

Dr. John Ottenweller, DVA Environmental Health Research Center, East Orange, N.J.

Dr. David Ozonoff, DVA Environmental Health Research Center, Boston, Mass.

MAJ Fred Peters, Department of Defense, Health Affairs, Washington, D.C.

Dr. Penny Pierce, University of Michigan, Ann Arbor

LTC Terry Rauch, MC, Office of Assistant Secretary of Defense, Washington, D.C.

Ms. Kathleen Scott, U.S. Air Force Office for Prevention and Health Services Assessment, Brooks AFB, Tex.

Dr. Linda Shortridge-McCauley, DVA Environmental Health Research Center, Portland, Oreg.

Dr. Fred Sidell, U.S. Army Medical Research Institute of Chemical Defense, Aberdeen Proving Ground, Md.

Dr. Peter Spencer, DVA Environmental Health Research Center, Portland, Oreg.

Dr. Steven Straus, National Institutes of Health, Bethesda, Md.

Dr. Robert Ursano, Uniformed Services University of Health Sciences, Bethesda, Md.

Dr. Bernard Wagner, National Academy of Sciences, Committee on Toxicology, Washington, D.C.

Dr. Roberta White, DVA Environmental Health Research Center, Boston, Mass.

Dr. Jessica Wolfe, DVA Medical Center, Boston, Mass.

Dr. Diana Zuckerman, staff to Senate Veterans Affairs Committee, Washington, D.C.

E

Other Groups Reviewing Persian Gulf War Veteran Health Issues

Board/Committee	Source of Funding	Nature of Activity	Status (May 1996)	Published Reports
PG Expert Scientific Panel	DVA	Provide advice to the VA on diagnosis, treatment, and research on PG-related health conditions	Ongoing	Periodic reports to the under secretary of the DVA
OTA Assessment of the DVA PGHR	Congress	Review of VA PGHR per PL 102-585	Completed	Report issued (U.S. Congress OTA, 1993)
OTA Review of DoD Kuwait Oil Fire Health Risk Assessment	Congress	Review of DoD Registry per PL 102-585	Completed	Report issued (U.S. Congress OTA, 1994)
Task Force on PGW Health Effects, Defense Science Board	DoD	Review reports of chemical, biologic, and toxic exposures in the PG	Completed	Report to the under secretary of Defense Acquisition (DSB, 1994)
PGVCB	DoD, DHHS, and DVA	Ensure interagency coordination of all efforts, separate and joint, in the areas of research, clinical care, and disability determination and compensation for post-ODS/S unexplained illnesses	Ongoing	PGVCB 1994, 1995a,b

RWG	DoD, EPA, DHHS, and DVA	Assess the state and direction of research, identify gaps in factual knowledge and conceptual understanding, identify testable hypotheses, recommend research directions for participating agencies, review research concepts as they are developed, and collect and disseminate scientifically peer-reviewed information	Ongoing	Annual report to Congress (PGVCB, 1995c; PGVCB RWG, 1996)
Disability and Compensation Working Group	DoD, DHHS, and DVA	Provide PGVCB sufficient data to make policy decisions on compensation for PG veterans	Ongoing	
Clinical Working Group	DoD, DHHS, and DVA	Provide PGVCB information regarding clinical care	Ongoing	
NIH Technology Assessment Workshop: The PG Experience and Health	Interagency	Develop a case definition of "mystery illness" and provide a list of recommendations	Completed	Report issued (NIH Technology Assessment Workshop Panel, 1994)
IOM Committee to Evaluate the DoD CCEP	DoD	Independent evaluation of the DoD's CCEP	Proposed to be extended	Report issued (IOM, 1996)

Continued

Board/Committee	Source of Funding	Nature of Activity	Status (May 1996)	Published Reports
PGW Veterans Illnesses Investigation Team	DoD	Investigate and analyze PG-illness-related classified and declassified material; respond to reports on incident "Hot Line" (800-472-6719)	Ongoing	Release of declassified data and posting of information on WWW at: http://www.dtic.dla.mil:80/gulflink/
Presidential Advisory Committee on Gulf War Veterans' Illnesses (PAC)	DoD	Executive Order 12961. Provide to the President, through the secretaries of DoD, DVA, and DHHS, advice and recommendations based on its review of PG research, coordinating efforts, medical treatment, outreach, external reviews, risk factors, and chemical and biological weapons	Ongoing	Interim report (PAC, 1996a); final report due Dec. 1996
IOM Committee to Evaluate the DVA UCAP	DVA	Independent evaluation of the VA's clinical protocols	Under development	

NOTE: CCEP = Comprehensive Clinical Evaluation Program; DHHS = Department of Health and Human Services; DoD = Department of Defense; DSB = Defense Science Board; DVA = Department of Veterans Affairs; EPA = Environmental Protection Agency; IOM = Institute of Medicine; NIH = National Institutes of Health; ODS/S = Operation Desert Shield/Storm; OTA = Office of Technology Assessment; PAC = President's Advisory Committee; PG = Persian Gulf; PGHR = Persian Gulf Health Registry; PGVCB = Persian Gulf Veterans Coordinating Board; PGW = Persian Gulf War; PL = Public Law; RWG = Research Working Group; UCAP = Uniform Case Assessment Protocol; VA = Veterans Administration; and WWW = World Wide Web.

F

Research and Related Activities on Health Problems of Persian Gulf War Veterans

Study	Investigator Affiliation or Study Center	Status (May 1996)
Mortality Studies		
Mortality follow-up study of PG veterans	VACO	Completed
Comparative Mortality Among U.S. Military Personnel Worldwide During ODS/S	WRAIR	Completed (Writer et al., 1996)
Hospitalization Studies		
Comparative study of hospitalizations among active duty military personnel	NHRC, San Diego, Calif.	Completed
Comparison of federal and nonfederal hospitalization rates among veterans who have separated from active service	NHRC, San Diego, Calif.	In progress
Studies of Self-Reported Symptoms: Outbreaks		
Investigation of a possible outbreak among ODS veterans at Fort Benjamin Harrison, Ind.	WRAIR	Completed (DeFraites et al., 1992)
Post-PG illness reported in Naval Reserve Mobile Construction Battalion 24	NEPMU No. 2, Norfolk, Va.	Completed

Continued

Study	Investigator Affiliation or Study Center	Status (May 1996)
CDC investigation of veterans in Pennsylvania	CDC	Phase I completed (MMWR, 1995); Phase II completed; Phase III In progress
Studies of Self-Reported Symptoms: Surveys		
National Health Survey of PG Veterans and Their Family Members	VACO	In progress
A study of symptoms among 1,500 Seabees—PG and era	NHRC, San Diego, Calif.	Completed
Seabee health study	NHRC, San Diego, Calif.	Submitted to OMB
Health Assessment of PGW Veterans from Iowa	Cooperative agreement between the CDC and University of Iowa, and the Iowa VAMC	In progress
Reproductive Health Studies		
A Comparative Study of Pregnancy Outcomes [Birth Defects] Among Gulf War Veterans and Other Active Duty Personnel	NHRC, San Diego, Calif.	Completed
Reproductive Outcomes in Gulf War Veterans	NHRC, San Diego, Calif.	In progress
Prevalence of congenital anomalies reported in state birth defects registries among children born to PGW veterans	NHRC, San Diego, Calif.	In progress

Study	Investigator Affiliation or Study Center	Status (May 1996)
Studies of Mental Health		
Stress-related surveys of active duty, guard, and reserve personnel	WRAIR, Dept. of Psychiatry	Completed (Marlowe, 1995; Marlowe et al., 1990a,b; WRAIR, 1992; Wright et al., 1991)
The General Well-Being of Gulf War Era Service Personnel from the States of Pennsylvania and Hawaii: A Survey	WRAIR, USAMRMC	Completed (USAMRMC, 1994; Stretch et al., 1995, 1996)
Desert Storm Reunion Survey	Boston, Mass., VAMC	Expanded (Wolfe et al., 1992c, 1993)
Early intervention with Appalachian Marine reservists in ODS	Mt. Home, Tenn., VAMC	Completed (Sloan et al., 1992; 1995a,b; 1996a,b)
Investigation of relation between experience in ODS and postwar adjustment	Clarksburg, W.Va., VAMC and Dept. of Psychology, W.Va. University	Completed (Scotti et al., 1993)
Psychological assessment of ODS returnees	New Orleans, La., VAMC	Expanded (Sutker et al., 1992, 1993, 1994a,b; 1995a,b)
Evaluation of Cognitive Functioning in PG Veterans Reporting War-Related Health Problems	New Orleans, La., and Boston, Mass., VAMC	In progress
Memory and Attention in PTSD	New Orleans, La., VAMC	In progress
Neuropsychological Functioning in Veterans	New Orleans, La., VAMC	Completed
Psychological adjustment in ODS/S veterans	Gainesville, Fla., VAMC	Completed (Sohler et al., 1992)

Continued

Study	Investigator Affiliation or Study Center	Status (May 1996)
ODS Outreach Program	Cincinnati, Ohio, VAMC	Completed (Baker et al., 1992)
West Haven VAMC ODS Report	West Haven, Conn., VAMC	Completed (Southwick and Morgan, 1992; Southwick et al., 1993)
The PG Outreach Program at the Little Rock VAMC	Little Rock, Ark., VAMC	Completed (Rodell et al., 1992)
An Evaluation of Troops Returning from the PG: A Preliminary Report	Providence, R.I., VAMC	Completed (Unger et al., 1992)
Coming Home for Good: The ODS Veterans and Family Psychosocial Debriefing Project	Portland, Oreg., VAMC	Completed (Ford et al., 1992)
PG Veterans Seen Through VA's Readjustment Counseling Service and Impact of the PGW on VA's Provision of Readjustment Counseling	Washington, D.C., VAMC	Completed (Blank and Gelsomino, 1992)
The Need for Continuing Mental Health Intervention in Soldiers Returning from the PGW: Assessment of Deployed and Nondeployed Reserve Units from Western Pennsylvania, Eastern Ohio, and West Virginia	Highland Drive, Pa., VAMC	Completed (Pontius et al., 1992)
Acute and long-term impact of deployment to SWA on the physical and mental health of soldiers and their families	USUHS and WRAIR	In progress
Combat Stress Diagnosis, PTSD prevention	USAMRMC and New Haven, Conn., VAMC	Ongoing
Women's Health Studies		
Health and Psychosocial Readjustment of Gulf War Women	U. Michigan School of Nursing	Completed (Pierce, 1995, 1996)

Study	Investigator Affiliation or Study Center	Status (May 1996)
Activation Experiences During the PGW	Beth El College of Nursing, Colorado Springs, Colo.; Air Wyoming Air National Guard, Cheyenne, Wyo.	Completed (Nelson et al., 1996)
VA EHRC		
East Orange, N.J.	East Orange, N.J., VAMC	In progress
Health and exposure survey of PG veterans		
Physiological and psychological assessments of PG veterans		
Effects of exertion and chemical stress on PG veterans		
Effects of genetics and stress on responses to environmental toxins		
Portland, Oreg.	Portland, Oreg., VAMC	In progress
Core Epidemiology Study		
Psychosocial, neuropsychological, and neurobehavioral assessment		
Clinical and neuroendocrine aspects of fibromyalgia		
Neurotoxicity of environmental pollutants and warfare agents		
DNA damage from chemical agents and its repair		
Boston, Mass.	Boston, Mass., VAMC	In progress
Evaluation of cognitive functioning of PG veterans		
Evaluation of neurological functioning in PG veterans		
Gulf War and Vietnam veterans cancer incidence surveillance		
Evaluation of respiratory dysfunction among Gulf War veterans		
The aromatic hydrocarbon receptor as a biomarker of susceptibility		
Validity of computerized tests		

Continued

Study	Investigator Affiliation or Study Center	Status (May 1996)
Environmental Studies		
Air-quality studies		
Kuwait Oil Fires: Interagency Interim Report	Interagency Air Assessment Team (EPA, DHHS, NOAA) and representatives from Coast Guard, DoD, and DoE	Completed (EPA, 1991)
Report to Congress: U.S. Gulf Environmental Technical Assistance (January 27–July 31, 1991)	International cooperative effort coordinated by UN; U.S. activities coordinated by EPA (PL 102-27)	Completed (U.S. Gulf Environmental Technical Assistance, 1992)
Human studies		
Report to Congress: Health Consequences of the exposure of PG Force members to the Fumes of Burning Oil	DoD	Completed (DoD, 1993)
Environmental toxicology studies	AFIP	Completed (AFIP, 1994; Moeller et al., 1994; Peterson and Kalasinsky, 1996)
Kuwait Oil Fire Health Risk Assessment	USAEHA (currently USACHPPM)	Completed (USAEHA, 1992, 1994)
Biologic Surveillance Initiative	USAEHA (currently USACHPPM); AFIP	Completed (USAEHA, 1994)
Animal studies		
Assessment of histopathological lesions and chemical analyses of feral cats to smoke from Kuwait oil fires	AFIP	Completed (Moeller et al., 1994)

Study	Investigator Affiliation or Study Center	Status (May 1996)
Physiological and neurobehavioral effects in rodents from exposure to PB, fuels, and DEET (toxicity of simulated PGW exposure)	USAMRMC	In progress
PB synergistic toxicity study	USAMRMC	Completed (USACHPPM, 1995)
Chronic organophosphorus exposure and cognition	Medical College of Georgia Research Institute	In progress
Evaluation of MWDs that participated in ODS/S	DoD Working Dog Center, Lackland AFB, San Antonio, Tex.	In progress
DU Research		
Health risk assessment of embedded DU: behavior, physiology, histology, and biokinetic modeling	AFRRI	In progress
Carcinogenicity of DU fragments	ITRI	In progress
Prophylactic Treatment Research		
A Study to Evaluate the Safety Tolerance, Pharmacokinetics, and Pharmacodynamics of PB	USAMRMC (contracted to the South Florida Research Corporation)	Completed (Lasseter and Garg, 1996)
Retrospective studies involving military use of pyridostigmine as pretreatment for nerve agent poisoning	USAMRICD	Completed
Possible relationship between multiple chemical sensitivity of DEET and carbamate (pyridostigmine) in PGW veterans' illnesses	WRAIR; WRAMC	In progress
Information Systems Activities		
GIS	USACHPPM	In progress
VA PGHR	VACO	Ongoing
VA PG Referral Centers	Washington, D.C.; Houston, Tex., West Los Angeles, Calif.; Birmingham, Ala.	Ongoing

Continued

Study	Investigator Affiliation or Study Center	Status (May 1996)
DoD CCEP	DoD MTFs	Ongoing
DoD SCC	WRAMC	Ongoing
Pilot Studies		
Risk Factors Among U.S. Army Soldiers for Enrolling on the VA PGHR	VACO; WRAIR	In progress
Extent of musculoskeletal problems associated with "GWS"	Long Beach, Calif., VAMC	In progress
Etiology of dyspnea occurring after PGW service	Washington, D.C., VAMC	In progress
Antibody testing for mycoplasma	WRAMC	Completed
Diarrhea in PG veterans: an irritable bowel–like disorder	Gainesville, Fla., VAMC	In progress
Clinical studies in PG veterans	Allen Park, Mich., VAMC	Ongoing
Post–Desert Storm miscarriage rates in six Army hospitals	U.S. Army, Office of the Surgeon General	Completed (Broadnax, 1992)
Birth defects and miscarriages in the families of PG veterans assigned to Robins AFB, Ga.	Robins AFB, Ga.	Completed (Eggert, 1994)
Spontaneous abortion rate and the Gulf War mobilization	William Beaumont Army Medical Center, Tex.	Completed (Rosa, 1993)
Children of PG veterans (624th quartermaster, 786 transportation)	Jackson, Miss., VAMC; CDC; Miss. State Health Department	Completed (Penman et al., 1996)
Retrospective survey of PG troops who received *Clostridium botulinum* toxoid	USAMMDA	Completed
Chronic Gastrointestinal Illness in Desert Storm Veterans: A Survey and Questionnaire	Boston, Mass., VAMC	In progress
A Preliminary Neuropsychological Study of PG Veterans	Highland Drive, VAMC; Pittsburgh, Pa.	Completed (Goldstein et al., 1996)
ODS: Activation, deployment and re-integration experiences of VAMC employees	Salt Lake City, Utah, VAMC	Completed (Allen et al., 1991)

Study	Investigator Affiliation or Study Center	Status (May 1996)
Supporting Research		
Leishmaniasis and infectious disease research		
Development of a leishmania skin test antigen	USAMRMC	Ongoing
Identification of the genetic factors that control tropism in *Leishmania*	DoD/VA	Ongoing
Vaccine-Mediated Immunity Against Leishmania	Cleveland, Ohio, VAMC	Ongoing
Serologic diagnosis of viscerotropic leishmaniasis	USAMRMC	Ongoing
Protective immunity in experimental visceral leishmaniasis	San Antonio, Tex., VAMC	Ongoing
Use of immunological techniques to study the interaction of carcinogens with DNA	NCI/NIH	Ongoing
Forward deployable diagnostics for infectious diseases	USAMRMC	Ongoing

NOTE: AFB = Air Force base; AFIP = Armed Forces Institute of Pathology; AFRRI = Armed Forces Radiation Research Institute; CCEP = Comprehensive Clinical Evaluation Program; CDC = Centers for Disease Control and Prevention; DEET = *N,N,*-diethyl-*m*-toluamide; DHHS = Department of Health and Human Services; DNA = deoxyribonucleic acid; DoD = Department of Defense; DoE = Department of Energy; DU = depleted uranium; EHRC = Environmental Health Research Center; EPA = Environmental Protection Agency; GIS = Geographical Information System; GWS = Gulf War Syndrome; ITRI = Inhalation Toxicology Research Institute; MTF = medical treatment facility; MWD = military working dog; NCI = National Cancer Institute; NEPMU = Navy Environmental and Preventive Medicine Unit; NHRC = Naval Health Research Center; NIH = National Institutes of Health; NOAA = National Oceanographic and Atmospheric Administration; ODS = Operation Desert Storm; ODS/S = Operation Desert Shield/Storm; PB = pyridostigmine bromide; PG = Persian Gulf; PGHR = Persian Gulf Health Registry; PGW = Persian Gulf War; PTSD = Posttraumatic stress disorder; SCC = Specialized Care Center; SWA = Southwest Asia; UN = United Nations; USACHPPM = U.S. Army Center for Health Promotion and Preventive Medicine; USAEHA = U.S. Army Environmental Hygiene Agency; USAMMDA = U.S. Army Medical Materiel Development Activity; USAMRICD = U.S. Army Research Institute of Chemical Defense; USAMRMC = U.S. Army Medical Research and Materiel Command; USUHS = Uniformed Services University of Health Sciences; VA = Veterans Administration; VACO = VA Central Office; VAMC = VA Medical Center; WMO = World Meteorological Organization; WRAIR = Walter Reed Army Institute of Research; and WRAMC = Walter Reed Army Medical Center.

G

Selected DoD, Army, Navy, Air Force, and DVA Databases

I. **DoD or Tri-Service**

A. **DMIS (Defense Medical Information System).** DMIS provides a large repository of patient level, normative, population and financial data to support the formulation and execution of plans, programs, and policies of the assistant secretary of defense (health affairs) and supports the information needs of the military departments' headquarters staff and health care analyses. DMIS is a centralized, non-deployed set of applications software and databases that support the collection, integration, validation, distribution, and analysis of MHSS data concerning population, cost, utilization, and medical treatment data.

B. **DMDC (Defense Manpower Data Center).** DMDC maintains central personnel databases.

C. **DMED (Defense Medical Epidemiological Database—under development).** Computer link of all relevant medical and personnel databases to describe population denominators. This is part of a tri-service effort to provide a means of sharing data between the military services and civilian companies for joint research studies. The Central Research Databases Project consists of several major tasks: identifying the data requirements of researchers in a variety of areas, such as epidemiology, occupational medicine, public health, preventive medicine, and medical readiness; developing a longitudinal, relational database for data, cross-mapping data between service branches; and developing user-friendly software to permit remote access to the Air Force and Navy data. Future databases will be added to provide TDY data, immunization and outpatient data, and other data of interest to the research community. A duty station location file will allow tracking of the individual's geographical location at any point in his/her career.

D. **WCRS (Worldwide Casualty Reporting System).** WCRS is a central repository of administrative reports (DD1300, Report of Casualty) of all active duty military deaths.

E. **MEPRS (USMEPCOM—Military Entrance Processing Reporting System, U.S. Military Entrance Processing Command).** MEPRS is a system with a database of all demographic, limited medical, aptitude tests and other administrative information on applicants to military service (i.e., includes those who do in fact enlist, as well as those rejected). The Army is the executive agent for this system.

F. **TEAM (Troop Exposure Assessment Model).** The TEAM is a database integrating GIS technology to incorporate USACHPPM air pollution data from the PG, NOAA modeling for the period of the burning oil well fires, satellite imagery of the geographic extent of the oil fire plumes, troop movement data, and PG exposure and toxicologic data as available.

G. **CCEP (Comprehensive Clinical Evaluation Program).** The DoD Comprehensive Clinical Evaluation Program (CCEP) provides a systematic, in-depth medical evaluation for DoD beneficiaries (Persian Gulf War veterans now on active duty or retired; members of the full-time National Guard who are Persian Gulf veterans; Persian Gulf War veterans who are members of the Ready Reserve/Individual Ready Reserve/Standby Reserve/Reserve who are placed on orders by their units; and eligible family members of such personnel) who are experiencing illnesses that may be related to their service in the Persian Gulf. Once a participant has completed the examination process, copies of examination results are forwarded to the CCEP Program Management Team (PMT), where they undergo quality assurance procedures, and the data are entered into the master CCEP database.

H. **ANSR (Army/Navy Serum Repository).** This repository is tied to the U. S. Army HIV Data System (USAHDS) maintained by USACHPPM. Database set up to track results of individual's HIV tests. The Serum Repository is a serum bank of all service members, maintained by the Army and Navy for sera stored since 1985.

I. **ACTUR (Automated Central Tumor Registry).** Provides uniformed services medical treatment activities with the capability for registration and tracking of cancer patients' records, course of treatment, outcomes, test results, and quality of life of the patient. ACTUR provides a single system to all DoD inpatient facilities for meeting the services standards, American College of Surgeons and state requirements for cancer programs. The database supports automated research capability and demographic reports.

II. **ARMY**

A. **AMSA (Army Medical Surveillance Activity).** The AMSA currently consists of four major components: a reportable disease surveillance system, the U.S. Army HIV data system (USAHDS), deployment medical surveillance, and acute respiratory disease surveillance. Future components of AMSA are to include disability data (USAPDA), health risk appraisals (HRAs), hospitalizations of active duty Army members in Navy or Air Force medical treatment facilities (MTFs), and Navy and Air Force reportable diseases.

B. **HRAs (Health Risk Appraisals).** Database of self-reported health-associated behaviors and attitudes and limited measures of health (blood lipids, blood glucose, blood pressure) for active duty soldiers, retirees, beneficiaries, and others.

C. **PARRTS (Patient Accounting and Reporting Real-Time Tracking System).** Automated medical information system that provides real-time in-bed visibility of contingency patients.

D. **IPDS (Individual Patient Data System).** Computerized inpatient record with eight discharge diagnoses, procedures, demographics, length of stay, and disposition.

III. **NAVY**

A. **CHAMPS (Career History Archival Medical and Personnel System).** CHAMPS is a Navy database with information maintained from the past 25 years. It has a medical outcome focus, with individual records containing chronological events.

B. **DMED (described above)**

C. **Inpatient Hospitalization Record.** Hospitalization database that is comparable to the IPDS, Air Force, and DVA's PTF hospitalization databases.

IV. **AIR FORCE (AF)**

A. **Inpatient hospitalizations.** Hospitalization database that is comparable to the IPDS, Navy, and DVA's PTF hospitalization databases.

B. **ASIMS (Aeromedical Services Information Management System).** The ASIMS is part of the medical surveillance data collection system, which has been fielded to all Air Force locations having a clinic or medical treatment facility. Data on cases of reportable diseases are collected and transmitted to a central repository. These data will be incorporated in the central research database.

C. **DMED (described above)**

V. **DVA (Department of Veterans' Affairs)**

A. **PTF (Patient Treatment File).** Inpatient hospitalization database similar to the three services.

B. **BIRLS (Beneficiary Identification Record Locator System).** Database of claims files, including death claims (verified by requesting copy of death certificate, which is put in the personnel record).

C. **NPCD (National Patient Care Database—under development).**

D. **PGHR (PG Health Registry).** Health examinations of PG veterans seeking the DVA's registry exam.

Acronyms

ACGIH: American Conference of Governmental Industrial Hygienists
AChE: acetylcholinesterase
ACTUR: automated central tumor registry
AF: Air Force
AFB: Air Force base
AFIP: Armed Forces Institute of Pathology
AFRRI: Armed Forces Radiobiology Research Institute
AIBS: American Institute of Biological Sciences
AIDS: acquired immunodeficiency syndrome
AMSA: Army medical surveillance activity
ANSR: Army/Navy serum repository
APA: American Psychiatric Association
ARCOM: Army reserve command
ASIMS: Aeromedical Services Information Management System
ATP: adenosine triphosphate

BAA: Broad Area Announcement
BIRLS: Beneficiary Identification and Records Locator Subsystem
BSI: Brief Symptom Inventory
BW: biological warfare

CARC: chemical-agent-resistant coating
CBW: chemical and biological warfare

CCEP: Comprehensive Clinical Evaluation Program
CDC: Centers for Disease Control and Prevention
CFS: chronic fatigue syndrome
CHAMPS: Career History Archival Medical and Personnel System
CHAMPUS: Civilian Health and Medical Program of the Uniformed Services
CI: confidence interval
CIA: Central Intelligence Agency
CNS: central nervous system
CW: chemical warfare

DDVP: dichlorvos
DEET: *N,N*-diethyl-*m*-toluamide
DHHS: Department of Health and Human Services
DISN: Defense Information System Network
DMDC: Defense Manpower Data Center
DMED: Defense Medical Epidemiological Database
DMIS: Defense Medical Information System
DNA: deoxyribonucleic acid
DoD: Department of Defense
DoE: Department of Energy
DSB: Defense Science Board
DSM: Diagnostic and Statistical Manual
DU: depleted uranium
DVA: Department of Veterans Affairs

EHRC: environmental hazards research center
EPA: Environmental Protection Agency

FDA: Food and Drug Administration
FEV1/FVC: ratio of forced expiratory volume in one second to forced vital capacity

GAO: General Accounting Office
GIS: geographical information system
GSI: General Severity Index
GWS: Gulf War Syndrome

HIV: human immunodeficiency virus
HPA: hypothalamic-pituitary-adrenal
HRA: Health Risk Appraisal

ICD-9: International Classification of Diseases, version 9
IES: Impact of Event Scale

IOM: Institute of Medicine
IPDS: Individual Patient Data System
IRR: Individual Ready Reserve
ITRI: Inhalation Toxicology Research Institute

MCS: multiple chemical sensitivity
MEPRS: Military Entrance Processing Reporting System
MFUA: Medical Follow-up Agency
MHSS: Military Health Surveillance System
MMWR: Morbidity and Mortality Weekly Report
MOPP: mission objective protective posture
MRE: meal, ready-to-eat
MRI: magnetic resonance imaging
MTF: medical treatment facility
MWD: military working dog

NAS: National Academy of Sciences
NASA: National Aeronautics and Space Administration
NCI: National Cancer Institute
NDI: National Death Index
NEPEC: Northeast Program Evaluation Center
NEPMU: Navy Environmental and Preventive Medicine Unit
NHRC: Naval Health Research Center
NIH: National Institutes of Health
NOAA: National Oceanographic and Atmospheric Administration
NPCD: National Patient Care Database
NRC: National Research Council

ODS: Operation Desert Storm
ODS/S: Operation Desert Shield/Storm
OMB: Office of Management and Budget
OPD: oxidative phosphorylation disorder
OPIDN: organophosphate-induced delayed neuropathy
OTA: Office of Technology Assessment

PAC: President's Advisory Committee
PAHs: polycyclic aromatic hydrocarbons
PARRTS: Patient Accounting and Reporting Real-Time Tracking System
PB: pyridostigmine bromide
PEL: permissible exposure level
PG: Persian Gulf
PGHR: Persian Gulf Health Registry
PGVCB: Persian Gulf Veterans Coordinating Board

PGVIIT: Persian Gulf Veterans Illnesses Investigation Team
PGW: Persian Gulf War
PL: public law
PMT: Program Management Team
PTF: Patient Treatment File
PTSD: posttraumatic stress disorder

RME: reasonable maximum individual exposure
RR: relative risk
RUL: Registry of Unit Locations
RWG: Research Working Group

SCC: Specialized Care Center
SCL-R-90: Symptom Check List-Revised-90
SCUD: Soviet-designed surface-to-surface missile
SWA: Southwest Asia

TAML: theater area medical laboratory
TDY: temporary duty
TEAM: Troop Exposure Assessment Model
TLV: threshold limit value
TRICARE: Regionalized tri-service health care system
TRI-SERVICE: Army, Navy, Air Force

UCAP: uniform case assessment protocol
UI: unexplained illnesses
UMR: uniform medical record
UN: United Nations
USACHPPM: U.S. Army Center for Health Promotion and Preventive Medicine
USAEHA: U.S. Army Environmental Hygiene Agency
USAHDS: U.S. Army HIV Data System
USAMMDA: U.S. Army Medical Materiel Development Activity
USAMRICD: U.S. Army Medical Research Institute of Chemical Defense
USAMRIID: U.S. Army Medical Research Institute of Infectious Diseases
USAMRMC: U.S. Army Medical Research and Materiel Command
USAPDA: U.S. Army Disability Database
USMEPCOM: U.S. Military Entrance Processing Command
USPHS: U.S. Public Health Service
USUHS: Uniformed Services University of Health Sciences

VA: Veterans Administration
VACO: VA Central Office

VAMC: VA Medical Center

WCRS: Worldwide Casualty Reporting System
WMO: World Meteorological Organization
WRAIR: Walter Reed Army Institute of Research
WRAMC: Walter Reed Army Medical Center